overcoming
high blood pressure

the complete complementary health program

Dr Sarah Brewer

In Association with The Complementary Medical Association

DUNCAN BAIRD PUBLISHERS

LONDON

Natural Health Guru: Overcoming High Blood Pressure

For my wonderful husband, Richard

First published in the United Kingdom and Ireland in 2008 by
Duncan Baird Publishers Ltd
Sixth Floor
Castle House
75–76 Wells Street
London W1T 3QH

Conceived, created and designed by Duncan Baird Publishers

Managing Editor: Grace Cheetham
Editor: Kesta Desmond
Managing Designer: Manisha Patel
Designer: Gail Jones
Typographical styling: Allan Sommerville
Commissioned artwork: Mark Watkinson
Commissioned photography: Toby Scott at Simon Smith studios
Styling: Mari Mererid Willliams
Picture research: Susannah Stone

British Library Cataloguing-in-Publication Data:
A CIP record for this book is available from the British Library

ISBN: 978-1-84483-381-8

10 9 8 7 6 5 4 3 2 1

Typeset in Univers
Colour reproduction by Scanhouse, Malaysia
Printed in China by Regent

Publisher's note: 1 tsp = 5 ml, 1 tbsp = 15ml, 1 cup = 250ml.
The information in this book is not intended as a substitute for professional medical advice and treatment. If you are pregnant or are suffering
from any medical conditions or health problems, it is recommended that
you consult a medical professional before following any of the advice or
practice suggested in this book. Duncan Baird Publishers, and any other
persons who have been involved in working on this publication, cannot
accept responsibility for any injuries or damage incurred as a result of
following the information, exercises, therapeutic techniques or recipes
contained in this book.

contents

high blood pressure introduction

High blood pressure is an insidious condition that creeps up on you with little warning. As a result, one in five adults has hypertension, yet at least half are unaware they are affected. This means an estimated one in 10 adults is walking around with an undiagnosed condition that can have serious effects on their long-term health – one in 10 of all your friends and relatives could be affected. Although you may have picked up this book for your own benefit please encourage everyone you know to have their blood pressure checked if they haven't done so in the past year – they may be surprised at the result.

When hypertension is diagnosed, treatment is important as high blood pressure hastens the hardening and furring up of your arteries, which increases blood pressure even more. It's a vicious circle that can, if uncontrolled, eventually lead to coronary heart disease, a stroke, impaired vision, kidney problems and poor circulation throughout your body – all from a condition that doesn't, in itself, make you feel unwell. Because high blood pressure is so potentially dangerous, it's important that it's monitored regularly and that you aim to keep your blood pressure below 130/80mmHg.

Although drugs are often needed to lower blood pressure, dietary and lifestyle changes can help bring down blood pressure significantly. In many cases, these changes mean you won't have to take anti-hypertensive medication at all. And, if you're already on drug treatment, dietary and lifestyle changes may lower your blood pressure enough for your doctor to start weaning you off the drugs you're taking.

This book provides all the information you need to help keep your blood pressure within safe limits. It gives you information about the important dietary and lifestyle changes you can make, why regular exercise is so important, the benefits of relaxation, and the natural health approaches that work. These approaches may be new to you. Rest assured that the information given is based on compelling clinical research. I have included only those complementary therapies, food supplements and dietary approaches that have the best possible chance of controlling your blood pressure naturally and safely.

Everyone is different and no diet and lifestyle plan will suit all individuals. For that reason, I've drawn up three different approaches: a gentle, a moderate and a full-strength program, one of which is likely to suit

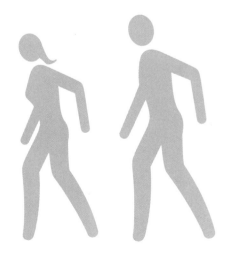

you. To help you work out which plan is right for you, answer the detailed questionnaire on pages 75–76. This will point you in the right direction.

For those who want to take things slowly, the gentle program introduces you to healthy eating principles such as cutting back on refined carbohydrates, cooking without salt, eating more fruit, vegetables and fish and lowering your consumption of red meat. Low doses of food supplements are also suggested. The gentle plan gets you stretching and walking, and introduces you to holistic complementary health approaches such as aromatherapy, homeopathy, meditation and yoga. The gentle program has the potential to lower your blood pressure by at least 4/2 to 7/4mmHg within 30 days.

For those who want more of a challenge, or who are already following a relatively healthy diet and lifestyle, the moderate program introduces you to a wider variety of wholegrains, bean sprouts and fruit and vegetable juices, and includes more of the superfoods shown to have beneficial effects on blood pressure. I suggest more therapeutic doses of supplements, and a more intensive exercise program. In addition, I introduce you to complementary approaches such as qigong, herbal medicine, reflexology and more advanced relaxation techniques. The moderate program has the potential to lower blood pressure by at least 7/4 to 11/5mmHg within 30 days.

For those who already eat healthily and are very physically active, I recommend the full-strength program. This includes a diet based on seven superfoods identified as having the most significant beneficial effects on circulatory health. Supplement doses are suggested at the higher end of the therapeutic range. I also introduce you to naturopathy, acupuncture and relaxation techniques such as transcendental meditation. The full-strength program has the potential to lower your blood pressure by at least 15/8mmHg over the course of just one month.

Look out for these symbols
Throughout this book I have included boxes that highlight useful, interesting or important pieces of information. Each box bears a symbol (see below). The arrow symbol indicates that a box contains practical instructions. The plus sign means the box contains additional information about the subject being discussed, or about high blood pressure in general. The exclamation mark indicates a warning or a caution.

This book takes a holistic approach, and is designed to complement the treatments your doctor prescribes. It is intended to offer general information, not to replace individual advice from your own doctor or other healthcare professionals who know your individual needs. Never stop taking your anti-hypertensive medication without your doctor's permission. Once your blood pressure starts coming down as a result of diet and lifestyle changes, your doctor should be happy to consider reducing your prescribed medication under careful medical supervision.

The information in this book is not intended for women who have high blood pressure during pregnancy. Never take food supplements or herbal remedies during pregnancy unless advised to by a doctor, pharmacist or qualified medical herbalist.

To accompany this book I have created a website: www.naturalhealthguru.co.uk. It features updated information, new recipes and the most recent research findings. Please visit the site regularly to tell me how you get on with the programs, and, most importantly, to share your successes.

Understanding high blood pressure

High blood pressure – or hypertension – can often be difficult to perceive as a serious medical condition. You may have been diagnosed with it, yet feel healthy. To fully understand high blood pressure, I think it helps to have some basic knowledge of the **workings of the heart and blood vessels**. In a healthy body blood pressure rises and falls throughout the day – a process that is facilitated by nerve signals, hormones and other chemicals. The **development of hypertension** means that instead of fluctuating normally, your blood pressure stays high all the time. I explain the two **different types of hypertension** and the risk factors associated with each. If you have hypertension, it's important to know about the **long-term complications**, such as coronary heart disease, so you can take action to prevent them, and be aware of their early signs and symptoms. The action you should take when you receive a **diagnosis of hypertension** depends on how high your blood pressure is – there are different categories that range from stage 1 (mild) to stage 3 (severe). Your doctor will decide whether you can manage your blood pressure through diet and lifestyle changes, or whether you need tablets. I describe the **range of medication** you might be offered, and explain how each treatment works.

what is blood pressure?

In order to function, all the tissues and organs in your body need a constant supply of oxygen and nutrients. These are supplied by your blood, which is pumped by your heart through a complex network of arteries and veins. The pressure at which your blood travels through your arteries is very important. If it is too high, it can damage or rupture a blood vessel, or result in bleeding in the brain. In the long term it can damage your organs. If blood pressure is too low, not enough blood – and therefore not enough oxygen and nutrients – reaches your body tissues and organs. If you've ever experienced low blood pressure as a result of standing up suddenly, you'll know that the main symptom is feeling faint. This is because the blood pressure in your arteries is temporarily too low to carry sufficient oxygen to your brain.

The rise and fall of blood pressure

I think it's helpful to compare the flow of blood through your blood vessels to the flow of water through a tube – a hosepipe, for example. The water pressure inside a hosepipe can vary from high to low, depending on factors such as how fully you turn on the tap or whether you constrict the hosepipe by squeezing it or inserting a blockage into it. The blood pressure inside your arteries rises and falls in a similar way. For example, if your heart beats faster and pumps out more blood, your blood pressure rises. If your blood vessels constrict or dilate, your blood pressure rises or falls respectively.

Your blood pressure fluctuates naturally throughout a 24-hour period. It is lowest when you are asleep (usually around 3am), and highest in the morning from the time before you awake to approximately 11am.

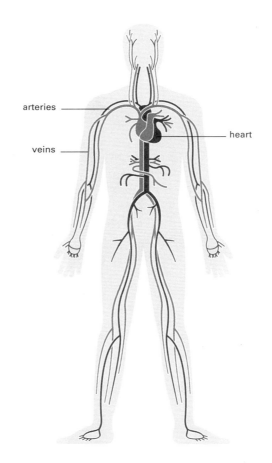

arteries

veins

heart

The cardiovascular system

The heart, arteries, veins and capillaries (the tiny blood vessels that connect arteries to veins) make up the cardiovascular system. The arteries are strong and flexible vessels that carry blood away from the heart at a relatively high pressure. Veins carry blood back to the heart at a lower pressure – they have thinner walls and larger diameters than arteries.

During your waking hours, your blood pressure goes up and down in response to a variety of factors. Anything that changes your cardiac output (the amount of blood that is pumped through your heart over a set period of time) will have an impact on your blood pressure. For example, exercise increases your cardiac output and causes your blood pressure to rise; so do anxiety, excitement, high environmental temperatures, eating and cigarette smoking. Obesity increases your cardiac output and therefore your blood pressure. Even drinking a cup of coffee can cause a temporary spike in your blood pressure.

These rises in blood pressure are completely normal – they are part of the daily rhythm of your cardiovascular system. Even if you run upstairs, go for a jog or encounter some highly stressful moments in your day, your body quickly restores your blood pressure to normal afterward. It is only when your cardiovascular system stops working properly (with age, for example) that high blood pressure becomes a problem – instead of rising and falling in a regular, predictable pattern it stays high all the time, even when you're sitting still. This permanent state of high blood pressure can damage your body and is known as hypertension (see pages 14–16).

Understanding blood pressure readings

Between each heartbeat your heart rests briefly. During this rest the upper chambers of your heart fill with blood, and your blood pressure is at its lowest point – this is known as diastole. Almost immediately afterward, your heart contracts to push blood out into your arteries. As a result, your blood pressure rises – this is known as systole.

When you have your blood pressure taken, the reading yields two numbers that are written one over the other: the first is your systolic blood pressure and the second is your diastolic blood pressure. Blood

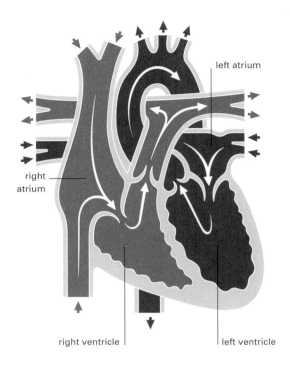

left atrium

right atrium

right ventricle   left ventricle

The chambers of the heart

When all the chambers of the heart relax, blood pressure is at its lowest. As the lower chambers of the heart (the ventricles) contract to force blood out of the heart, blood pressure is at its highest.

pressure is measured in millimetres of mercury, which is abbreviated to mmHg (Hg is the chemical symbol for mercury). So if you have a blood pressure reading of 120/80mmHg, this means your systolic pressure is 120 and your diastolic pressure is 80. When spoken, this is usually expressed as "one twenty over eighty". This reading is typical for a healthy adult at rest, though a blood pressure of 130/80mmHg is also considered acceptable. See page 20 for more information about how blood pressure is measured.

Structures in your heart and blood vessels, called baroreceptors, play an important role in monitoring your blood pressure. They detect how stretched your blood vessels are.

When your heart works harder to pump blood round your body (when you lift a heavy weight or during exercise, for example), it's your systolic pressure that tends to rise. However, as your arteries age and lose their elasticity (as happens in hypertension), it's your diastolic pressure that tends to creep up.

The normal control of blood pressure

To understand what goes wrong when you have hypertension, it's helpful to know how the healthy body normally regulates blood pressure. These are the main mechanisms:

- Altering the speed and force at which your heart contracts so that more or less blood is pumped into your circulation.
- Relaxing or constricting your blood vessels (to vary the amount of blood they hold).
- Regulating the volume of blood in your circulation by altering the amount of salt and fluids filtered out by your kidneys.
- Regulating the volume of blood in your circulation by triggering feelings of thirst, which then prompt you to drink.

These control mechanisms are partly regulated by nerve signals from your central nervous system, and partly by hormones and related substances released from various parts of your body including your kidneys, adrenal glands, pituitary gland and heart.

Baroreceptors: the body's blood pressure monitors

In the walls of your heart and blood vessels are structures called baroreceptors. These play an important role in monitoring your blood pressure. They work by detecting how stretched your blood vessels are (the greater the pressure your blood exerts on your vessel walls, the more they stretch).

understanding high blood pressure

If your blood pressure rises and your blood vessels stretch, your baroreceptors are more highly stimulated than usual. This sets in action a chain of events that causes your blood pressure to fall: your heart rate slows, your blood vessels dilate and the secretion of blood-vessel constricting chemicals decreases. When your baroreceptors detect a fall in blood pressure (for example, when you go from lying down to a standing position), they trigger an increase in your heart rate. They also trigger the prompt increase of an important hormone called renin (see below). Signals constantly pass between your baroreceptors and your brain to keep your blood pressure at a normal level.

The renin-angiotensin system Renin is a hormone that is produced by your kidneys and released into your bloodstream. It sets off a chain reaction that culminates in the rise of your blood pressure. Renin acts on a substance in the blood called angiotensin. As a result, angiotensin I is produced.

Angiotensin I, in turn, is quickly acted upon by angiotensin-converting enzyme (ACE) to form angiotensin II. Angiotensin II causes your arteries to constrict rapidly, which raises both your systolic and diastolic blood pressures. Angiotensin II is one of the most powerful blood vessel constrictors known. One of the mainstays of high blood pressure treatment is a group of drugs that block angiotensin-converting enzyme. These are known as ACE inhibitors (see page 24). Another type of drug that is prescribed for hypertension is beta-blockers – among other actions, these lower blood pressure by decreasing the body's secretion of renin.

As well as causing your arteries to constrict, angiotensin II triggers feelings of thirst (drinking increases the volume of fluid in your body and therefore your blood pressure). It also increases the secretion of two hormones: anti-diuretic hormone and aldosterone. Both of these help raise blood pressure.

The role of anti-diuretic hormone Anti-diuretic hormone, also known as vasopressin, is released by your brain's pituitary gland when prompted to by angiotensin II. It acts on your kidneys to decrease urine production. This means that more fluid stays in your body, which helps to raise your blood pressure.

The role of aldosterone Aldosterone is a steroid hormone secreted by your adrenal glands. It increases the reabsorption of sodium (in exchange for potassium) from your urine, sweat, saliva and intestinal juices. This draws fluid back into your body to help increase blood volume and raise blood pressure.

One rare cause of secondary hypertension (the less common type; see page 16) is the excessive production of aldosterone by the adrenal glands. This is known as Conn's syndrome.

The role of natriuretic hormone The other important hormone in blood pressure regulation is natriuretic hormone, which is secreted by the heart. In contrast to the hormones mentioned above, natriuretic hormone lowers blood pressure. It does this by inhibiting the secretion of renin from the kidneys and increasing the excretion of sodium and water. It also inhibits the secretion of anti-diuretic hormone from the pituitary gland in the brain.

Low blood pressure
Some people have blood pressure that is too low – known medically as hypotension. The symptoms are dizziness and fainting. Hypotension may be caused by heart problems, taking certain drugs or excessive fluid loss from the body as a result of diarrhoea or major bleeding from an injury.

what is hypertension?

Hypertension is the medical term for high blood pressure. If you have hypertension, your blood pressure is high all the time – even when you are at rest. People may wonder if the words "hyper" and "tension" imply a nervous, hyper or tense personality. The answer is no: "hypertension" refers strictly to elevated blood pressure rather than temperament.

Although hypertension is usually symptomless, it can pose a serious threat to your long-term health if you don't manage it by making changes to your diet and lifestyle, or by taking medication prescribed by your doctor.

For 90 percent of people with high blood pressure, no obvious single cause is identified. They are described as having primary or essential hypertension. For the other 10 percent of people, an identifiable cause is discovered – these people are referred to as having secondary hypertension.

Hypertension and scar tissue
An interesting predictor of whether someone will develop hypertension is the way in which their body forms scars. Some people produce an excessive amount of scar tissue in response to injury and have large, lumpy scars. These people are twice as likely to develop hypertension compared with those who produce normal scar tissue. The link between scar tissue and hypertension appears to be angiotensin II (see page 13); as well as raising blood pressure, angiotensin II stimulates production of collagen – the fibrous protein found in scar tissue.

Essential hypertension
The exact cause of essential hypertension remains unknown, but it's thought to result from an interaction between inherited, developmental and lifestyle factors.

Inherited factors Your genetic make-up influences how well your body is able to control your blood pressure. Genes can affect:

- The sensitivity of your baroreceptors (see page 12) and your renin-angiotensin system (see page 13)
- The responsiveness of your blood vessels to signals that tell them to dilate or constrict.
- How well your kidneys are able to flush excess sodium and fluid from your circulation.
- How an amino acid called homocysteine is processed by your body. Abnormal homocysteine processing results in a blood pressure rise of 0.7/0.5mmHg in men and 1.2/0.7mmHg in women for each 5 micromole per litre increase in circulating homocysteine concentrations. If homocysteine builds up, it hastens the development of atherosclerosis (see page 15), which also contributes to the development of hypertension.

Developmental factors An inadequate diet during pregnancy can affect the way the circulatory system forms in the developing embryo. It has been found that low birthweight babies are more likely to go on to develop hypertension as adults. Researchers have found that average adult systolic blood pressure increases by 11mmHg as birthweight goes down from 3.4kg (7½lb) to 2.5kg (5½lb). The highest blood pressures occur in men and women who were born as small babies with large placentas. Poor nutrition during your early development also affects your fingerprint patterns (which form arches, loops or whorls). Adults with one whorl have a blood pressure that is 6 percent higher than in those with no whorls, and blood pressure increases as the number of whorls increase (the maximum number is 10: two per digit) with most people having two or three.

Lifestyle factors Scientists now know that lifestyle factors interact with inherited factors to predispose certain people to hypertension in later life. These lifestyle factors include:

- Smoking cigarettes.
- Consuming excess salt in your diet.
- Drinking too much alcohol.
- Stress.
- Lack of exercise.
- Poor nutrition.
- Following a high-glycemic index diet (see page 54).
- Obesity.
- A low intake of vitamins B6, B12 and folic acid. (This increases your likelihood of developing hypertension if your ability to process the amino acid homocysteine is poor.)

The good news is that, even if you are genetically or developmentally predisposed to high blood pressure, you can take steps to prevent or delay its onset – this book will show you how.

Atherosclerosis This is the hardening and furring of the arteries that happens naturally with age, but which is hastened by many of the risk factors described above. Atherosclerosis is a main cause of high blood pressure. As arteries lose elasticity, the walls become

increasingly hard and rigid. They also "fur up" – fatty deposits, known as atheromas, are laid down on the lining of the artery walls. Hard arteries can no longer dilate effectively, and furred arteries make the flow of blood slower because the diameter of the artery is narrowed. The combined effect is a rise in dystolic

Furred-up arteries
As people get older, their arteries tend to lose flexibility. Not only do arteries become more rigid, they also get furred up with fatty deposits. This is called atherosclerosis and it is both a cause and an effect of hypertension.

Healthy artery

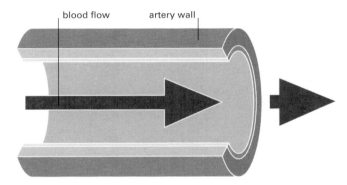

blood flow   artery wall

Artery affected by atherosclerosis

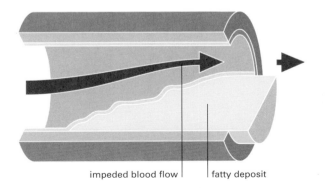

impeded blood flow   fatty deposit

blood pressure. Conversely, high blood pressure can also hasten atherosclerosis (see page 15). It does this by putting the artery walls under excessive strain.

Secondary hypertension

Hypertension that has a single major underlying cause is known as secondary hypertension.

Kidney disease In 80 percent of cases of secondary hypertension, the cause is a kidney (renal) disease that prevents excess fluid and salts being filtered from the body properly. They build up in the circulation and raise blood pressure. The kidneys also secrete an increased amount of renin hormone (see page 13), which contributes to the development of hypertension.

Pregnancy Around one in 10 pregnant women experience a type of secondary hypertension known as pre-eclampsia. This usually resolves after childbirth.

Drug side-effects Some drugs, including some over-the-counter drugs, can cause secondary hypertension. These include non-steroidal anti-inflammatory drugs (for example, ibuprofen), which can raise blood pressure by 5–10mmHg; the combined oral contraceptive pill which, after several years' use, increases blood pressure by an average of 2.8/1.9mmHg; ephedrine (a nasal decongestant); prednisolone (an oral corticosteroid); monoamine-oxidase inhibitors (an older type of antidepressant that causes sudden rises in blood pressure when eating specific foods); and carbenoxolone (sometimes used to treat stomach ulcers), which encourages the retention of sodium and water.

Rare causes Although rare, secondary hypertension can be caused by the following:

- Anatomical abnormalities (such as congenital narrowing of the aorta or renal artery).
- Excess production of red blood cells (polycythaemia), which increases blood volume and stickiness.
- Excess production of aldosterone hormone (Conn's syndrome).
- Excessive exposure to corticosteroids (Cushing's syndrome).
- Excess production of growth hormone (acromegaly).
- Excess production of parathyroid hormone (hyperparathyroidism).
- A rare type of adrenal gland tumour (phaeochromocytoma).

The symptoms of hypertension

When blood pressure rises temporarily in a healthy person – during exercise, for example – there are few, if any, symptoms (some people feel a pounding in their ears). There is often the same lack of symptoms in hypertension. Even if symptoms do occur, they tend to be non-specific, such as headache or passing urine more often at night. The latter symptom occurs when hypertension is linked with fluid retention – lying down at night causes excess fluid to be redistributed and filtered out by the kidneys.

It is only when blood pressure is severely raised that you get more specific symptoms such as dizziness, visual disturbances or the occasional nosebleed. This is why regular blood pressure checks are so important.

Your homocysteine level
A raised homocysteine level is linked with damage to the arteries, and an increased risk of heart attack and stroke. Make sure you know your homocysteine level – ask your doctor for a test or buy a home test.

complications
of hypertension

Although hypertension is often symptomless, it's vital to treat it, because, unchecked, it can lead to life-threatening illnesses such as kidney problems, eye disease, coronary heart disease, stroke and peripheral vascular disease. Even if you don't yet have these complications, you should be aware of them.

Kidney problems

The role of the kidneys is to filter the blood and to rid your body of waste products in the form of urine. The kidneys also maintain a healthy amount of fluid and salts in your body. In the long term, high blood pressure can lead to the hardening and furring of the arteries that supply the kidneys. It can also damage small blood vessels inside the kidneys. As a result, the kidneys receive a poor supply of blood and they may:

- Start to shrink (atrophy).
- Function less well and produce less urine.
- Leak protein into the urine (this is an important sign of many early kidney diseases).

Damage to the kidneys is often symptomless. In fact, by the time you start to experience symptoms – such as swollen ankles, shortness of breath, itchy skin and nausea – your kidneys have already lost a significant amount of their filtering ability. At this point you will be losing protein into your urine. If damage continues, your kidneys will produce progressively less urine, and waste products and fluid will remain in your body. The late symptoms of kidney disease include swelling of the abdomen, face and limbs, weight loss, vomiting and severe lethargy.

Kidney damage is usually diagnosed by a variety of urine and blood tests. At first, kidney damage may be managed by tight control of your blood pressure. You may be prescribed medication to reduce the amount of protein you lose in your urine. During the later stages of kidney damage, treatment may consist of dialysis or a kidney transplant. Dialysis involves artificially filtering your blood, sometimes with a dialysis machine.

Damage to the kidneys

If the renal artery that supplies the kidneys becomes hard and narrow, the kidneys may be damaged by an inadequate blood supply. High blood pressure in the tiny blood vessels inside the kidney can also damage the kidney's filtering units – the nephrons.

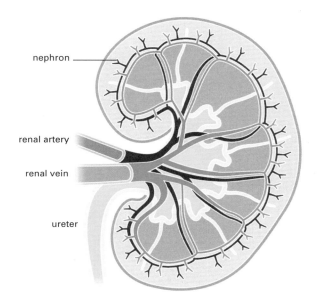

nephron

renal artery

renal vein

ureter

Eye disease

Over time, hypertension can damage the small blood vessels in the retinas at the back of the eyes. This is known as hypertensive retinopathy. In the early stages of retinopathy, your vision is unaffected. However, in later stages of retinopathy, your vision may be reduced and, in severe cases, you may have partial or complete sight loss. Hypertension is usually diagnosed and treated before it becomes this severe.

People with high blood pressure should have regular eye examinations to check for signs of damage to the retina. Retinal changes are divided into the following stages of severity:

● ●

Damage to the retina

The retina is the area at the back of the eye that receives light. Like other blood vessels in the body, the retinal blood vessels are susceptible to damage by hypertension. If the damage is unchecked, this can lead to a loss of vision.

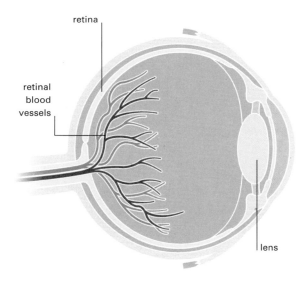

retina

retinal blood vessels

lens

- ● Grade one: the retinal arteries appear thickened and bulging.
- ● Grade two: the arteries compress the veins where they cross.
- ● Grade three: the arteries leak blood and fluid.
- ● Grade four: the optic nerve swells and bulges.

If grade three retinal changes are diagnosed, your hypertension urgently needs to be controlled. Grade three changes are associated with a similar level of deterioration to the blood vessels in the brain – this puts you at risk of a stroke (see page 19). You may be asked to stay in hospital until your hypertension is under control.

Coronary heart disease (CHD)

Over time, high blood pressure can hasten the development of a condition called atherosclerosis (see page 15) in which the arteries become hard, and narrowed with fatty deposits known as atheromas. (It can also work the other way round; atherosclerosis can lead to high blood pressure.)

If your coronary arteries are affected by atherosclerosis, the blood flow to your heart is less efficient. As damage progresses, your heart may receive an insufficient supply of oxygen and this may lead to the symptoms of coronary heart disease, which are described below.

Coronary heart disease may be treated with either tablets or surgery. Surgery may include coronary artery bypass surgery or coronary angioplasty. Bypass surgery involves grafting a blood vessel from another part of your body to divert blood away from the damaged section. Angioplasty involves widening the artery by inserting a fine tube into the artery. A balloon on the tip of the tube is inflated inside the blocked section, then deflated and withdrawn. The symptoms of coronary heart disease are as follows:

Angina This refers to a sensation of pain or pressure in your chest that comes and goes. It usually occurs when you are stressed or when you exert yourself. You may also experience pain in your left shoulder or on the inside of your left arm.

Heart attack This is a sudden pain in the chest that may be accompanied by breathlessness, a pounding heart, sweating, nausea and light-headedness, and sometimes loss of consciousness. Heart attack symptoms are sometimes relatively mild.

Heart failure The heart, rather than failing completely as the name of this condition would suggest, gradually loses its ability to pump blood around your body. This leads to swelling in your legs, feet and abdomen, severe tiredness and breathlessness.

Stroke

If atherosclerosis affects the flow of blood to your brain, you are at risk of a blood clot, or a leakage of blood into the brain (as a result of a burst vessel). If this happens, you have a stroke. Your brain is deprived of oxygen and brain cells in the affected area are damaged or die. The symptoms of a stroke depend on which part of your brain has been damaged. Your vision, speech, memory, hearing, movement or balance may be affected.

The treatment of a stroke consists of helping you recover the functions that were lost or damaged. For example, you might receive physiotherapy to restore movement or speech therapy to help you talk again.

Peripheral vascular disease

Peripheral vascular disease occurs when the arteries in your legs and arms become narrowed by fatty deposits that restrict the flow of blood. Because blood cannot get through, your leg muscles are prone to cramping,

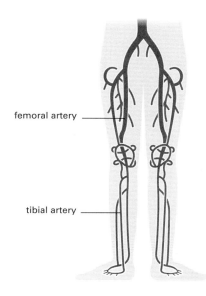

femoral artery

tibial artery

Blood supply to the legs
The legs need a plentiful supply of blood from the arteries to enable muscles to work properly. If the flow of blood is restricted, the muscles start to cramp and movement is impeded.

• •

especially during physical activity when their demand for blood and oxygen increases. In severe cases, just walking a short distance on flat ground can cause cramping. In very severe cases, pain may even occur when you are sitting down. Peripheral vascular disease is most likely if you have hypertension and you are a smoker, or if you also have diabetes.

Peripheral vascular disease can also make it difficult for men to achieve or maintain an erection because narrowed arteries mean blood supply to the penis is reduced.

The treatment for peripheral vascular disease consists of tablets or surgery – either bypass surgery or angioplasty; see page 18.

diagnosis and screening

Your blood pressure may rise from year to year, which is why it's important to monitor it regularly. As you get older, you should have your blood pressure checked at least once every three years, and preferably annually.

Blood pressure is checked using a sphygmomanometer. This consists of a cuff that is attached to a digital blood pressure monitor. The cuff is wrapped around your upper arm and inflated to a high pressure, which stops blood from flowing to your lower arm. As the cuff is slowly deflated, the monitor reads your systolic and diastolic blood pressure (see page 11).

If you're diagnosed with hypertension, you will be described as having stage 1, 2 or 3 hypertension. It may be possible to treat stage 1 hypertension with lifestyle changes, but the other two stages are usually treated with medication in combination with lifestyle changes. See pages 22–25 for more about treatment.

white-coat hypertension

A doctor usually takes your blood pressure several times before diagnosing hypertension. This is because your blood pressure may be high on one occasion but

What your blood pressure reading means

blood pressure reading	classification	treatment
120/80mmHg	Optimal	No treatment necessary (though always adopt a healthy lifestyle).
130/80mmHg	Normal	Reassess in five years and adopt a healthy lifestyle.
130/80–139/89mmHg	Pre-hypertension	Reassess yearly (treat if there is high risk of heart disease).
140/90–159/99mmHg	Stage 1 hypertension (mild)	If no complications, no diabetes and a low risk of cardio-vascular problems, monitor blood pressure every two to three months and reassess risk of cardiovascular disease annually. If complications, diabetes or a high risk of cardiovascular disease, treat with medication. In both cases, make lifestyle changes.
160/100–179/109mmHg*	Stage 2 hypertension (moderate)	Treat with medication and lifestyle changes.
180/110mmHg	Stage 3 hypertension (severe)	Treat with medication and lifestyle changes.

* Or a sustained diastolic blood pressure of equal to or above 100mmHg, despite diet and lifestyle measures.

no on the next – some people feel so anxious about the experience of visiting the doctor or having their blood pressure taken that it causes a rise in their blood pressure. This is known as "white-coat hypertension". White-coat hypertension, which may increase systolic blood pressure by 20–30mmHg, is suspected when a person has a normal blood pressure when they check it at home, but a high reading in the presence of a doctor.

If there is doubt about a diagnosis of hypertension, a doctor may recommend that your blood pressure is monitored over a 24-hour period, using an ambulatory monitoring device. This consists of a cuff that is attached to a monitor by a tube. The cuff, which you wear around your arm for 24 hours, inflates and deflates at intervals to measure your blood pressure.

Screening for complications

If you're diagnosed with hypertension, your doctor will want to find out whether you have developed any of the complications associated with high blood pressure (see pages 17–19) such as coronary heart disease or eye disease. For example, he or she may look for signs of excess fluid in your body (this can be a sign of heart failure) by pressing on the skin of your lower limbs to see if this leaves a pit. He or she will also listen to your heart and lungs using a stethoscope. Other tests that may be carried out are:

Eye examination The retinas at the backs of your eyes may be damaged by high blood pressure – this is called hypertensive retinopathy. Your doctor can check for this by looking into your eyes with an instrument called an ophthalmoscope. The health of the blood vessels in the backs of your eye, can provide useful information about the health of your cardiovascular system in general. For example, one 2006 study confirmed that having retinopathy is linked with double the risk of heart enlargement and stroke.

Urine test High blood pressure can damage your kidneys. Your urine will be tested for the presence of substances that may indicate kidney damage.

Chest x-ray An x-ray reveals the size and shape of your heart. It can also detect heart failure, which is a symptom of coronary heart disease.

Electrocardiogram (ECG) This measures the rhythm and electrical activity of your heart. It can show how high blood pressure has affected the working of your heart and whether you have had a heart attack.

Blood tests Your blood is tested for the levels of fats such as cholesterol and triglycerides – high levels of some fats (see page 51) increase your risk of coronary heart disease. Your blood level of an amino acid called homocysteine is also assessed. High homocysteine promotes atherosclerosis (see page 15) and abnormal blood clotting. As many as one in 10 heart attacks and strokes may be attributable to raised homocysteine, making it at least as important a risk factor as high cholesterol. Your blood will also be tested for glucose and salt (sodium, potassium and chloride) levels.

Interpreting homocysteine levels

homocysteine level	risk level
6.9micromol/L	Optimum (low risk)
7–9.9micromol/L	Mild risk
10–12.9micromol/L	Moderate risk
13–20micromol/L	High risk
Above 20micromol/L	Very high risk

treating hypertension

The early diagnosis and treatment of hypertension is important to reduce the risk of the complications described on pages 17–19. Once your doctor has established that you have hypertension, he or she will recommend that you make a number of lifestyle changes. Depending on your stage of hypertension (see page 20), he or she may also prescribe drugs. Blood pressure treatment aims to bring your systolic blood pressure to 140mmHg or below and your diastolic blood pressure to 90mmHg or below. If you have coronary heart disease (CHD) or are at high risk of it, a lower target of 130/80mmHg is recommended.

Adjusting your lifestyle

A doctor will encourage you to make the following diet and lifestyle changes. These can help you avoid drug treatment, or they can complement the blood pressure-lowering effects of medication, perhaps enabling you to reduce the dose or number of drugs you need.

- Eat at least five servings of fresh fruit and vegetables per day (see pages 49–50).
- Reduce your intake of unhealthy fat, such as saturated fat (see pages 51–52).
- Reduce your salt intake to less than 6g (1/5oz) sodium chloride or less than 2.4g (2/25oz) sodium per day (see page 53).
- If you smoke, quit (see page 66).
- Limit your alcohol intake to three or fewer units a day if you are a man, or two or fewer units a day if you are a woman (see page 67).
- Find coping strategies to help you deal with stress.
- Take regular aerobic exercise, such as brisk walking, for at least 30 minutes a day, ideally on most days of the week (see page 69).
- Lose weight if you need to. Then maintain a healthy weight for your height (see pages 70–71).

Drug treatments

If your blood pressure is elevated to a level that requires drug treatment, your doctor will select one or more medications from the following classes. These drugs are taken in tablet or capsule form and are known as anti-hypertensives.

- Thiazide diuretics.
- Beta-blockers.
- Calcium channel blockers.
- ACE inhibitors.
- Angiotensin II blockers.
- Renin inhibitors may also become available.

Monitoring hypertension
When you have hypertension it is important to monitor your blood pressure at home. Self-inflating upper arm and wrist monitors are validated as accurate, though the measurements you obtain are typically lower than those measured by a doctor – probably because you are more relaxed at home. A home measurement of less than 130/80mmHg is considered optimal. If possible, buy a monitor with a memory so you can record your readings at the same time of day every week. Your doctor can then download the information.

Your medication is a crucial investment in your future health. Together with lifestyle changes, it reduces the risk of life-threatening conditions such as stroke and coronary heart disease.

Because hypertension is unlikely to make you feel ill on a day-to-day level, it can be frustrating to have to take tablets. However, your medication is a crucial investment in your future health. Together with diet and lifestyle changes, it reduces the risk of life-threatening conditions such as stroke and coronary heart disease.

People often ask how long they must take anti-hypertensives for. Although many people have to take them for life, this is not inevitable. It may be possible to stop taking anti-hypertensives if you don't have any complications of hypertension, and if you successfully lower your blood pressure by adopting the diet and lifestyle measures on the opposite page. However, it is important that once you start taking a drug, you don't make any changes without consulting your doctor. If your doctor decides you can lower the dose of your medication, or stop taking it all together, he or she will decrease the dose in a gradual stepwise fashion. This is necessary to avoid a sudden increase in your blood pressure.

In my opinion, the way to get the best from anti-hypertensive drugs is to take a close interest in your blood pressure (see the box opposite on monitoring hypertension). If you notice that your blood pressure is not responding to a new drug, or an increase in the dose of a drug, ask your doctor to review your treatment. On the other hand, if your home monitoring reveals that your blood pressure is coming down (thanks to losing weight, for example), ask your doctor about the possibility of lowering your dose.

Thiazide diuretics Thiazide diuretics lower your blood pressure by increasing the loss of salts and fluid through your urine. They typically act within one to two hours of taking them. For this reason it is better to take them in the morning rather than at night so that you won't need to get out of bed to empty your bladder. At first, you may notice that you are urinating more

Secondary hypertension

If you are thought to have secondary hypertension (the less common type of hypertension), you will be tested for the possible underlying causes and these will be treated appropriately. Your blood will be tested for levels of hormones that control blood pressure, such as aldosterone, cortisol and renin. Your blood or urine will also be assessed for levels of substances that, if raised, are known to cause hypertension. For example, a high level of vanillylmandelic acid may indicate a tumour of the adrenal glands. You will also have an ultrasound scan of the kidneys or other kidney tests – this is because kidney disease is the most common underlying cause of secondary hypertension.

often than usual. This wears off after the first few days because thiazides also encourage the mild dilation of small arteries so fluid in your circulation is redistributed. High doses of thiazides are avoided as they can lead to sodium/potassium imbalances. Thiazide diuretics are often prescribed to older people who also have heart failure. They are not prescribed if you have gout, as they can aggravate this condition.

Beta-blockers Beta-blockers lower blood pressure in the following ways:

- Decreasing the workload of your heart by slowing your pulse to around 60 beats per minute and reducing the force of each heartbeat.
- Reducing the sensitivity of baroreceptors (blood pressure sensors in the walls of your heart and blood vessels; see page 12).
- Altering the way blood vessels dilate or constrict.
- Blocking the effects of the stress hormone adrenaline.

- Lowering the secretion of a kidney hormone, renin (see page 13).

If beta-blockers need to be stopped, the dose is usually tapered off gradually so your blood pressure does not suddenly increase (known as rebound hypertension). Beta-blockers are best avoided in people with asthma as they can trigger an attack. Their most troublesome side-effects include fatigue, cold extremities and problems with sexual function. A beta-blocker is ideal for someone with angina or who has previously had a heart attack. However, in general there is a move away from using beta-blockers for hypertension.

Calcium channel blockers Calcium channel blockers slow the movement of calcium into your muscle cells. This reduces the force of contraction of the heart, relaxes arteries, reduces arterial spasm and allows peripheral veins to dilate so they hold more blood. Side-effects can include flushing, headache, ankle swelling and constipation. A calcium channel blocker is often selected for older people who have a raised systolic blood pressure, but a relatively normal diastolic blood pressure, or who have angina. In the UK there is a general move towards using calcium channel blockers (and ACE inhibitors) as a first-line treatment option in preference to thiazide diuretics or beta-blockers.

ACE inhibitors One of the body's most powerful ways of increasing blood pressure is the renin-angiotensin system (see page 13), which involves angiotensin-converting enzyme (ACE). Drugs that block the action of this enzyme (ACE inhibitors) prevent the production of angiotensin II – a powerful blood vessel constrictor. Small arteries and veins are therefore able to dilate, causing blood pressure to fall. By increasing blood flow to your kidneys, this class of drug also encourages the loss of water and sodium in your urine.

Because ACE inhibitors can cause a sudden fall in blood pressure with the very first dose, treatment is often started at night on retiring to bed. One of the most troublesome side-effects of the drug is a persistent dry cough. An ACE inhibitor is often selected for people who also have heart pump failure. In the UK there is a general move towards using ACE inhibitors (and calcium channel blockers) as a first-line treatment option in preference to thiazide diuretics or beta-blockers.

Angiotensin II blockers Angiotensin II blockers are similar to ACE inhibitors, but they work one step further on, in that they block the formation of angiotensin II (see page 13). The end result is the same: dilation of arteries and veins, increased blood flow to the kidneys and increased production of urine. Interestingly, angiotensin II blockers may also act on the central nervous system to reduce thirst so you drink less. Side-effects of these drugs, such as dizziness, are usually mild.

Other anti-hypertensive drugs Some other anti-hypertensive drugs are used in special cases, such as pregnancy. In addition, another group of drugs called alpha-blockers (for example, doxazosin, indoramin, prazosin and terazosin) are mainly reserved for use in men who have urinary symptoms due to an enlarged prostate gland – alpha-blockers help shrink the prostate gland as well as reducing blood pressure.

Additional drugs that may be prescribed In addition to anti-hypertensive drugs, your doctor may decide it is beneficial for you to take other drugs. These may include statin drugs, which lower the level of unhealthy cholesterol in your blood (as with hypertension, high cholesterol is a risk factor for cardiovascular disease). Aspirin is also sometimes prescribed because of its ability to prevent abnormal blood clotting.

How drugs are prescribed

Your doctor will select the most appropriate drug for you depending on your age and whether you have complications.

The lowest recommended dose of the drug is prescribed.

This often produces an effect within 24 hours, but your full response to the drug is monitored over at least four weeks (unless your blood pressure needs lowering urgently).

After four weeks the dose of the drug is slowly increased according to the manufacturer's instructions.

If the increase doesn't adequately control your blood pressure, a second or third drug is added.

If your blood pressure remains too high, another drug is added.

The natural health approach In this section I explain how you can lower your blood pressure using **complementary therapies**, and making dietary and lifestyle changes. These tools can not only lower your blood pressure, but can also **improve your overall health and well-being**. In many cases, these natural approaches to treatment work so well that your doctor may wish to reduce the number or dose of drugs you are taking. The complementary therapies in this section are all **safe and effective** for people with hypertension – some, such as aromatherapy, reflexology and yoga can lower blood pressure by relaxing you, while others, such as acupressure, acupuncture and herbal medicine, work on a deeper level. Perhaps one of the most exciting approaches is that of **dietary change**: relatively simple steps such as cutting back on your salt intake; consuming more fruit, vegetables, fish and garlic; eating superfoods such as almonds; and even enjoying small amounts of red wine and dark chocolate have the power to transform your health. Key **nutritional supplements** can also have a positive impact on your blood pressure. Finally, I look at how **changing your lifestyle** can help you. Taking more exercise, maintaining a healthy weight, not smoking, enjoying alcohol in moderation and reducing stress can literally add years to your life.

complementary approaches to treatment

The holistic approach to treating hypertension includes a number of complementary therapies that you can use in conjunction with the drugs your doctor prescribes. In many cases, you will benefit from visiting a therapist, at least at first.

If you have pre-hypertension or mild hypertension (see page 14) and are not yet taking medication, it's likely that complementary approaches, together with dietary and lifestyle changes, will lower your blood pressure to a point at which you won't need drugs. If you are already taking medication to treat hypertension, it's important to continue taking your drugs alongside any therapies you try. That's why therapies are best referred to as complementary rather than alternative therapies – they *complement* medical treatment rather than providing a true alternative. Another phrase used to describe the combined use of orthodox and complementary therapies is "integrative medicine", which, essentially, cherry-picks the best approaches.

Which therapies can help?

Over the next few pages, I give an overview of the main complementary therapies that can help hypertension: aromatherapy, naturopathy, herbal medicine, homeopathy, reflexology, acupuncture, yoga, qigong and meditation. Some approaches, such as aromatherapy, yoga and meditation, work mainly through relaxation and overcoming stress, while others, such as homeopathy, reflexology and acupuncture harness your body's natural healing abilities to lower your blood pressure. In contrast, herbal medicine uses plant extracts that have a physiological effect in the body, modifying its function in a similar way to some drugs.

Consulting a therapist

It's important to consult a properly qualified practitioner, who is accredited with the appropriate umbrella organization, and who carries indemnity insurance. Most umbrella organizations provide lists of qualified practitioners who are registered with them. Many also have a facility on their website to help you find a therapist in your area. Some useful addresses are provided in the resource section on pages 174–175.

Having checked the qualifications of your chosen therapist, ask about their experience and successes in treating hypertension. Find out how long a course of treatment is likely to last, and the likely cost, before committing yourself to an appointment.

Having consulted a therapist, you may find you need only one or two consultations – for example, with a homeopath or medical herbalist – to point you in the right direction and enable you to use that therapy at home. With other therapies, such as reflexology, yoga and aromatherapy massage, you may decide to attend regularly for on-going practitioner-led benefits.

Always tell your therapist that you have hypertension, and which, if any, prescribed medications you are taking. If your blood pressure starts coming down as a result of a therapy, tell your doctor. He or she should be happy to slowly reduce the number or dose of the drugs you are taking.

aromatherapy

The main principle of aromatherapy is that inhaling specific scents can change your physiological state. This happens because smell has an important impact on your brain – in particular on a primitive part of your brain called the limbic system that helps regulate memory, arousal, emotions and hormone secretion. The scents used by aromatherapists are essential oils derived from plants. Depending on the particular plant, the essential oil may be harvested from the flowers, leaves, seeds, roots, fruits or wood.

Essential oils are highly concentrated plant extracts and should be used with care (see the guidelines below right). They are almost always diluted with a "carrier" oil such as avocado, almond, calendula, grapeseed, jojoba or wheatgerm oil before they are used. Dilution is important because neat essential oils can irritate the skin and may have adverse effects – some can even raise blood pressure. One of the few exceptions to the dilution rule is lavender essential oil, which is often used neat. It's also acceptable to use essential oils neat when you're not applying them to the skin, for example, when adding them to a candle-lit diffuser to produce a therapeutic atmosphere.

In the case of hypertension, essential oils can help by relaxing you, promoting sleep, and making you less anxious – all of which help lower your blood pressure. Some essential oils lower blood pressure in other ways, for example, by having a diuretic action on the body, which means they flush out excess fluids.

Oils for treating hypertension

If you visit an aromatherapist, he or she will assess your health and choose a blend of essential oils that are suited to your particular needs. He or she will probably massage the diluted oils into your skin and you may be given an ointment or lotion, or essential oil blend, to take home with you. Your aromatherapist will give you specific instructions about how to use any essential oil product. For more information about consulting an aromatherapist, see page 174.

You can also use aromatherapy as a self-help treatment at home. I suggest you select one, two, three or four essential oils from the chart on page 30. Base your choice on both the therapeutic effects of the oils and your personal scent preferences. If you choose a scent you really like, you'll relax more easily. How you blend the oils together is also a matter of personal taste. Experiment until you find a scent blend you particularly like. If a blend isn't quite to your liking, add more drops of one or more of the oils – or introduce another that you feel might be missing. Keep a note of the total

Guidelines for using essential oils

- Do not take essential oils internally.
- Before using an essential oil blend on your skin, put a small amount on a patch of skin and leave it for an hour to ensure you are not sensitive to it.
- Do not use essential oils if you are pregnant, or likely to be, except under specialist advice from an aromatherapist.
- Keep essential oils away from your face and eyes.
- If you are taking homeopathic remedies, do not use peppermint, rosemary or lavender essential oils as they may neutralize the homeopathic effect.
- Essential oils are flammable, so do not put them on an open flame.
- Avoid thyme, clove and cinnamon essential oils, which can raise blood pressure.
- Always keep essential oils out of the reach of children.

number of drops you use so that you can dilute it with the correct amount of carrier oil and recreate it again in the future. You can add an essential oil blend to a bath, massage it into your skin or diffuse it in the atmosphere.

When buying essential oils, look for the words "pure essential oil" on the label, rather than "aromatherapy oil". Products with the latter label may contain only small amounts of essential oils and will not have the same therapeutic effect.

Aromatherapy baths Select a blend of up to three essential oils. Add 5 drops of the blend to 10ml of a carrier oil and mix. Draw your bath so it's a comfortable temperature, then add the aromatic oil mix once the taps are turned off. Close the bathroom door to keep in the vapours and soak in the bath for 15–20 minutes, preferably in candlelight. Lie back comfortably and close your eyes. Allow the scent to fill your entire body and imagine it coursing through your blood vessels, bringing deep relaxation and lowering your blood pressure. At the end of your bath, dip a wet sponge in the oil mix on the surface of the water and use it to gently massage your whole body before rinsing.

Massage An oil blend intended to come into contact with your skin for massage should contain a maximum total of 1 drop of essential oil per 24 drops of carrier oil. This equates to 5 drops of essential oil in 10ml of carrier oil. It can help to buy a 5ml medicinal teaspoon or a 5ml syringe from a pharmacy to ensure accuracy – kitchen teaspoons tend to hold less than 5ml. You can massage parts of your body such as your legs and feet by yourself, but for a relaxing whole body massage, recruit a friend or partner.

Oil burners Using an oil burner is a good way to administer essential oils at night to help you sleep. Add 2 or 3 drops of a relaxing blend (for example, lavender or lemongrass blended with neroli) to a little warm water over a burner. Let the relaxing oils diffuse into your bedroom before retiring (make sure the candle is snuffed out before you get into bed). Alternatively, add 2 or 3 drops to a tissue and tuck it under your pillow. Another technique, which I recommend for use in the daytime, is to add a few drops of essential oil to a piece of cotton wool. Place this in a small sealed vial or plastic box, then open and inhale it at intervals throughout the day.

Essential oils that can help hypertension

relaxing and calming oils	oils to promote sleep	diuretic oils for hypertension with fluid retention	oils to help essential hypertension
Camomile, cedarwood, clary-sage, geranium, jasmine, juniper berry, lavender, lemon, lemongrass, melissa, neroli, orange, petitgrain, rose, sandalwood, ylang ylang	Camomile, clary-sage, geranium, juniper berry, lavender, lemongrass, melissa, neroli, orange, petitgrain, rose, sandalwood, ylang ylang	Camomile, cedarwood, geranium, juniper berry, lemon, peppermint, pine	Clary-sage, lavender, lemon, marjoram, melissa

naturopathy

Naturopathy is based on the belief that the body can find its own healthy equilibrium given the right conditions, such as a healthy diet, plenty of sleep, regular exercise and relaxation, fresh air, a clean environment, a stress-free lifestyle, plus a positive mental attitude.

A naturopath will work with you to help you reach this state of healthy equilibrium. He or she will use a variety of approaches including dietary changes, supplements, biochemic tissue salts, herbal remedies, homeopathy, hydrotherapy, massage, reflexology, relaxation techniques (including yoga) and sometimes physical manipulation. Many naturopaths are trained in iridology (a system of diagnosis involving examination of the iris of the eye), kinesiology (a system of diagnosis based on muscle strength), hypnotherapy, osteopathy, chiropractic or psychotherapy. Skin brushing, water sprays or friction rubs are often used to stimulate skin function and to boost the circulation.

The importance of diet

Naturopathic dietary approaches involve following a wholefood, high fibre – and preferably organic – diet that concentrates on fresh and, preferably, raw foods. A naturopathic diet is ideal for someone with hypertension as it's low in salt and fat, high in fibre and antioxidants, and contains plenty of fruits, vegetables, nuts, seeds, wholegrains and pulses. For hypertension, garlic and onions are recommended, together with foods rich in potassium, calcium and magnesium (alfalfa, avocados, broccoli, carrots, celery, lima beans, mushrooms, spinach and most fruits). Mineral water (eight glasses per day) is crucial to eliminate wastes, and a naturopath will usually advise you to avoid caffeine. Supplements of antioxidants (vitamins C and E), magnesium, potassium, co-enzyme Q10 and omega-3 fish oil may be recommended, together with herbal remedies.

Biochemic tissue salts

Naturopaths also use homeopathic remedies based on inorganic salts. These are known as biochemic tissue salts and are considered vital for health – depletion of any particular salt causes illness. Although biochemic tissue salts are prepared in the same way as homeopathic remedies, their use is very different; whereas the usual principle of homeopathy is "like treats like", tissue salts are given to correct a mineral deficiency. You may be prescribed calc. fluor for hypertension, or kali phos to relieve anxiety and stress.

Sleep and mental well-being

Naturopathy emphasizes the importance of sleep. Research suggests that lack of sleep increases activity in the sympathetic nervous system, which can increase blood pressure and pulse rate. Stress reduction is also important. In a study of people with mild to moderate hypertension, 70 percent of those who practised relaxation reduced their medication after six weeks, and within a year, 55 percent required no medication.

Naturopaths also place great importance on a positive state of mind to help overcome ill health. Interesting research shows that smiling boosts immunity. And hugging family and friends has been shown to produce warm feelings due to release of the hormone oxytocin, which is involved in bonding. Oxytocin has been shown to lower blood pressure by slowing the heart rate at times of stress, especially in women.

Daily naturopathic exercises
Breathe slowly and deeply, so air enters the bottom of your lungs, for two minutes twice a day. Before your daily bath or shower, brush your skin with a loofah or skin brush to improve circulation.

herbal medicine

Herbal medicine is one of the most ancient complementary therapies. In fact, more than 30 percent of medically prescribed drugs are derived from traditional plant remedies, such as aspirin (from the willow tree and meadowsweet plant), morphine (from opium poppy) and digoxin (from foxglove).

Whereas prescribed drugs contain a single active ingredient that is often manufactured synthetically, herbal supplements contain a blend of natural constituents that have evolved together in synergistic balance. This tends to produce a gentler action with less risk of side-effects.

Different parts of different plants are used in herbal medicine – roots, flowers, leaves, bark, fruit or seeds – depending on which has the highest concentration of active ingredients. The relevant part of the plant is usually harvested and made into an infusion (also known as a tea or tisane). Plants can also be dried and ground to produce a powder. This powder can be made into an infusion, an alcohol solution (also known as a tincture) or tablets/capsules. Modern technology also allows the extraction of active ingredients to produce more concentrated remedies.

Herbs for treating hypertension

A wide range of herbal remedies are effective for treating hypertension and associated problems, such as atherosclerosis. If you consult a medical herbalist, you may be prescribed one of the herbs I describe below. You can also buy or make your own herbal remedies. If I provide dosage information about one of the following herbs, the herb is safe to take without supervision. However, please read the warning in the caution box on page 33 before taking any herbal remedies.

Garlic (*Allium sativum*) Garlic is one of the most effective herbal remedies for people with hypertension. Research shows that it can reduce the risk of heart disease and stroke by 50 percent. It provides a number of beneficial substances including allicin (diallyl thiosulphinate), ajoene, methylallyl trisulphide and dimethy trisulphide. It has been found to reduce levels of cholesterol and triglycerides (see page 51) in the blood by around 12 percent after four months of taking it. Garlic also decreases blood stickiness, which makes the formation of clots less likely (hypertension is linked with an increased risk of blood-clotting and stroke).

Other research shows that garlic can lower blood pressure by dilating small arteries and veins by 4–6 percent, and by improving the elasticity of major arteries. These changes mean the heart has to work less hard to pump blood into the circulation. Garlic has even been shown to reverse atherosclerosis (see page 15) by decreasing the volume of fatty deposits on artery walls. In one study lasting four years, the volume of fatty deposits in the arteries was found to decrease by 15.6 percent in people taking garlic tables, while people taking an inactive placebo experienced a 2.6 percent increase in the volume of fatty deposits.

In combination, all of these effects can lower resistance in your arteries so that your blood pressure falls. A daily dose of 600–900mg garlic can reduce systolic blood pressure by an average of 8 percent (and by up

Making a herbal infusion
Infusions are made in a similar way to tea. Take a handful of the freshly picked herb (mint or lemon balm, for example) and place it in a warmed glass or china teapot. Cover with boiling water and leave to infuse for 10 minutes, then strain into a mug and drink.

to 17 percent), and reduce diastolic blood pressure by an average of 12 percent (and up to 16 percent) within two to three months of treatment. Include garlic in your diet as much as possible (add it near the end of cooking for maximum benefits). Consider taking a daily garlic tablet, too. *Dose:* Select tablets standardized to provide 1000–1500mcg allicin daily.

Hawthorn (*Crataegus oxycantha* and *Crataegus monogyna*) Hawthorn flowers and berries can lower blood pressure by relaxing the blood vessels in the peripheral circulation and improving blood flow to the heart muscle by dilating the coronary arteries. It also blocks the action of angiotensin-converting enzyme in a similar way to ACE inhibitor drugs (see pages 24–25). Other benefits include a mild diuretic action, which helps lower blood pressure by flushing excess fluid and sodium from the circulation. Hawthorn also has a calming effect that helps counteract stress. Hawthorn increases the strength and efficiency of the heart's

pumping action in people with heart failure (see page 19). Only take hawthorn under the supervision of a medical herbalist.

Dandelion (*Taraxacum officinalis*) Dandelion is good for hypertension that is linked to water retention. It has a diuretic action that helps to flush excess water and sodium from the body through the kidneys – but only in people with fluid retention. If your water balance is normal, dandelion does not have a diuretic action. *Dose:* 500mg extracts twice a day. Do not take dandelion if you have active gallstones or obstructive jaundice.

Lemon balm (*Melissa officinalis*) Lemon balm leaves are used during stressful times for their calming properties. Known as the "scholar's herb", lemon balm is widely recommended for exam stress. Herbalists use

Drinking lemon balm tea can help relieve the effects of stress, improve heart function and lower blood pressure.

When to avoid taking herbs
Do not take herbal remedies during pregnancy or when breastfeeding, unless you are specifically advised to by a medical herbalist or doctor. If you're taking any prescribed drugs, consult a qualified herbalist or pharmacist before taking a herbal remedy.

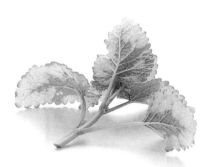
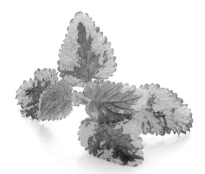
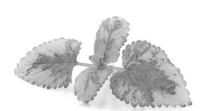

Valerian can help lower blood pressure during times of stress. It's one of the most relaxing herbs available. In one trial its effects were almost as strong as a prescription tranquillizer.

it to improve heart function and lower blood pressure. Try drinking tea containing lemon balm for its soothing effects. *Dose*: 650mg three times a day.

Bilberry (*Vaccinium myrtillus*) Bilberries contain purple antioxidant pigments called anthocyanidins that have been shown to strengthen small blood vessels, especially in the eye. One of the complications of high blood pressure is a deterioration in eyesight caused by retinopathy (see page 18). In some cases, taking bilberry extracts can improve visual acuity by 80 percent within two weeks. Blueberries provide similar anthocyanidins to bilberries but in smaller concentrations (as their flesh is cream-coloured rather than purple), but it's still worth including blueberries and their juice in your diet. *Dose:* 80–160mg bilberry extract, three times daily.

Artichoke (*Cynara scolymus*) Unhealthily high cholesterol levels often accompany hypertension and contribute to the development of cardiovascular problems. Artichoke extracts reduce cholesterol levels by decreasing the synthesis of cholesterol in the liver, and by increasing the conversion of cholesterol to bile acids. *Dose*: 320mg capsules, 1–6 daily with food.

Kudzu (*Pueraria lobata*) Also known as Japanese arrowroot, kudzu is a rich source of isoflavone plant hormones. Studies suggest that drinking kudzu root tea daily can have a significant impact on hypertension. Kudzu can also be used to help you reduce your alcohol intake. *Dose:* 150mg three times a day.

Bugleweed (*Lycopus europaeus*) Bugleweed is used to treat heart failure (a complication of hypertension). The aerial parts of the plant increase the contracting power of the heart, dilate blood vessels, reduce heart rate and have a diuretic action. Take bugleweed only under the supervision of a medical herbalist.

Chrysanthemum (*Chrysanthemum morifolium*) Flowers from this species of chrysanthemum are used in traditional Chinese medicine to improve coronary circulation, to increase the pumping action of the heart and to reduce and stabilize hypertension. Take chrysanthemum only under the supervision of a medical herbalist.

Lime blossom (*Tilia europea*) This is used medicinally to lower blood pressure and promote relaxation. It contains antioxidant flavonoids plus a natural sedative that relieves tension and promotes sleep. Drink an infusion of lime blossom in the evening before bedtime (you can make your own infusion or buy herbal teabags that blend lime blossom with other beneficial herbs).

Mistletoe (*Viscum album*) Mistletoe is used by herbalists to regulate blood pressure in both hypertension and hypotension. It's often combined with hawthorn (see page 33) in the treatment of hypertension. Take it only under the supervision of a medical herbalist.

Motherwort (*Leonurus cardiaca*) Leaves from the motherwort plant can strengthen the heart muscle, reduce palpitations, regulate a rapid pulse rate and lower hypertension. Take it only under the supervision of a medical herbalist.

Valerian (*Valeriana officinalis*) Valerian contains natural sedatives that make it one of the most relaxing herbs available. In one trial its sedative effects were almost as strong as a prescription tranquillizer. It's widely used to relieve anxiety, reduce stress, induce sleep and lower blood pressure, especially when high blood pressure is linked to excessive stress. Try drinking teas containing valerian for its soothing effects. *Dose*: 250–800mg, two to three times daily. Select products that are standardized to provide at least 0.8 percent valeric acid.

Standardization of herbal products

During the production of commercial herbal remedies, a small sample from each batch is taken.

The amount of one or two important active ingredients in the sample is measured.

The batch is then either diluted or concentrated so that a standard amount of active ingredient is present in the finished product.

If you choose a "standardized" herbal product, you can be sure you will receive a consistently effective dose. Standardized remedies are also more likely to have clinical trials supporting their use.

homeopathy

Homeopathy was founded around 200 years ago by the German physician Samuel Christian Hahnemann (1755–1843). It is based on the belief that tiny amounts of natural substances can stimulate the body's own healing powers. The term "homeopathy" literally means "similar suffering", and natural substances are selected that, if used at full strength, would trigger the same symptoms they are designed to treat. In minuscule homeopathic doses, however, the opposite effect occurs, and symptoms improve. This is the first principle of homeopathy: like cures like.

The second major principle of homeopathy is that less cures more. This describes the observation that increasing the dilution of a solution increases its potency. So, by diluting noxious substances many millions of times, their healing properties are enhanced and their undesirable side-effects are lost.

How homeopathy works is not completely understood, but contact with the original remedy is believed to polarize water molecules so they retain a unique electromagnetic signature. This is thought to have a dynamic action that boosts your body's own healing power.

Homeopathic treatments

Homeopathic remedies are made from plant, animal or mineral extracts that are chopped or ground, then steeped and shaken in an alcohol/water solution for two to four weeks. This mixture is strained into a dark glass bottle to produce the concentrated mother tincture, from which dilutions are made.

Homeopathic tablets are made by adding a few drops of these solutions to lactose (milk sugar) pillules and swirled together. The lactose tablets are stored in airtight, dark glass bottles, out of direct sunlight. Take homeopathic remedies in the following way:

- Tip the pill into your mouth from the lid of the bottle or from a spoon (don't handle it).
- Suck or chew the pill – don't swallow it whole.
- Don't eat or drink for 30 minutes before or after taking a remedy.
- Avoid strong tea or coffee, or powerful essential oils such as rosemary and peppermint. These may diminish the effect of homeopathic remedies.
- If symptoms worsen initially, persevere. This is a sign that the remedy is working.
- If there is no improvement, tell your homeopath – you may need a different remedy.

How effective is homeopathy?

Clinical trials have shown that homeopathy is significantly better than an inactive placebo in treating many chronic conditions, including hayfever, asthma, migraine, skin problems and rheumatoid arthritis. Some research has shown that two homeopathic remedies, Baryta carbonicum and Crataegus, can lower systolic and diastolic blood pressure in some people, though results from other studies were less convincing. Homeopathy seems to work best for those with early or borderline hypertension, who are not yet taking medication, or who are on only one anti-hypertensive drug.

Consulting a homeopath

Although you can buy your own homeopathic remedies, I advise visiting a homeopath for treatment that is individually tailored. A homeopath will select your treatment based not just on your symptoms, but also on your constitution, personality, lifestyle, family background and tastes. For more information about consulting a homeopath, see page 175.

After completing a course of homeopathy, you will usually feel better in yourself with a greatly improved sense of well-being that allows you to cope in a generally more positive way.

Homeopathic remedies for hypertension

remedy	prepared from	used to treat
Baryta carbonicum	Barium carbonate crystals	Headaches; cardiovascular problems, including hypertension
Baryta muriaticum	Barium chloride crystals	Hypertension with a high systolic and low diastolic pressure
Adrenalinum	Adrenaline (epinephrine) hormone	Sustained stress
Glonoinum	Glyceryl trinitrate	Hypertension associated with sudden flushing or increased blood flow to the head
Serum anguillar icthyotoxin	Eel serum	Hypertension associated with fluid retention and kidney problems
Thyroidinum	Dried sheep/calf thyroid gland	Hypertension associated with being overweight
Nux vomica	Strychnine-containing seeds of the poison nut	Intermittent arterial hypertension; stress associated with overwork and lifestyle excesses (smoking, eating or drinking too much)
Crataegus	Hawthorn	Hypertension, irregular pulse or heart failure (gives heart and circulatory support)
Passiflora incarnata	Passion flower	Stress (it calms and soothes the nervous system)
Picric acidum	Picric acid	Headaches; stress due to overwork; fatigue; fluid retention
Phosphoricum acidum	Phosphoric acid	Listlessness; stress due to bad news; lethargy
Ignatia	Seeds from St Ignatius' bean tree	Headache; stress following emotional upset
Arnica montana	Leopard's bane plant (sneezewort)	Emotional shock; abnormal blood clotting

reflexology

Reflexology is believed to originate from India, China and Egypt, and date back more than 5,000 years. It was first practised in the West by Dr William Fitzgerald in 1913 (he called his technique "zone therapy"). His work was developed further in the 1930s by Eunice Ingham to create what we now know as reflexology. Reflexology relaxes the body, mind and spirit, improves circulation and normalizes bodily functions. Its aim is to treat the symptoms and the causes of illness.

According to reflexology theory, points on the feet and hands – known as reflexes – relate to internal organs, structures and their function. These reflexes are represented as maps on the surfaces of the feet and the hands (though most reflexologists work on the feet). The right foot corresponds to the right side of the body, and the left foot to the left side of the body. Reflexes are present all over the foot – on the soles, upper foot, toes and ankles.

· ·

Reflexes on the soles of the feet

These are simplified reflexology diagrams showing some of the foot reflexes that correspond with major body organs. If you have hypertension, a reflexologist is likely to work on your heart, thyroid, spine and kidney reflexes. He or she may also work on your chest reflexes, which are on the top of your feet.

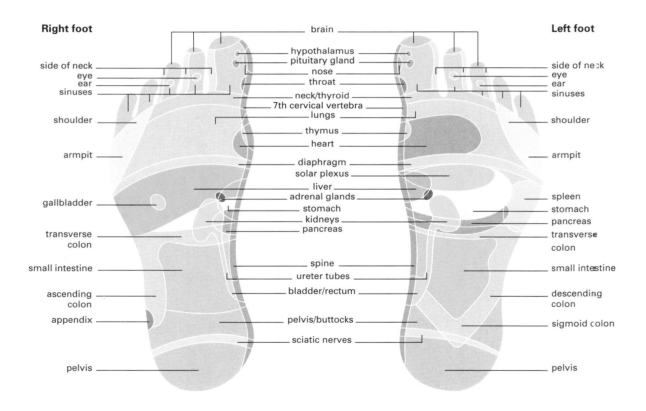

Right foot

- side of neck
- eye
- ear
- sinuses
- shoulder
- armpit
- gallbladder
- transverse colon
- small intestine
- ascending colon
- appendix
- pelvis

brain
hypothalamus
pituitary gland
nose
throat
neck/thyroid
7th cervical vertebra
lungs
thymus
heart
diaphragm
solar plexus
liver
adrenal glands
stomach
kidneys
pancreas
spine
ureter tubes
bladder/rectum
pelvis/buttocks
sciatic nerves

Left foot

- side of neck
- eye
- ear
- sinuses
- shoulder
- armpit
- spleen
- stomach
- pancreas
- transverse colon
- small intestine
- descending colon
- sigmoid colon
- pelvis

How effective is reflexology?

Reflexology is said to work best for disorders of the internal organs and for stress-related problems such as headache. A survey carried out by the Association of Reflexologists in the UK found that stress and hypertension were the conditions most successfully treated by its members.

Consulting a reflexologist

A therapist massages your feet using firm thumb and finger pressure. He or she also treats specific problems by applying pressure to appropriate reflex points. This stimulates nerve endings that pass from your feet to your brain and then to the relevant part of your body.

While massaging your feet, a therapist may also come across points on your feet that are unusually tender. By observing which bodily organs these points are related to, it is possible to diagnose health problems you may not be aware of. A reflexologist can treat these problems by working on the tender spots.

To treat hypertension, a reflexologist will typically concentrate on your heart reflex, which stretches from the diaphragm line (see diagram opposite) toward the base of the toes on both feet. Massaging the heart reflex on your left foot is said to strengthen and regulate your heart, while concentrating on the diaphragm line helps deepen your breathing and bring more oxygen into your body.

On the sole of your foot, at the base of your big toes, is the reflex area for the thyroid and parathyroid glands. Stimulating these helps to regulate your pulse rate and calcium metabolism, which can have a positive effect on your blood pressure. Finally, your spinal reflex, on the inside edge of both feet, is massaged to support your nervous system. Massaging the kidney areas (located at the top of your arches) helps flush excess fluid from your body. At the end of each session, you should feel warm, contented and relaxed.

Self-help reflexology

Although I recommend consulting a reflexologist for professional and individually tailored treatment, you may also benefit from massaging the reflexes in your foot yourself. To do this, familiarize yourself with the position of the diaphragm line, which stretches across the ball of each foot. The following massage will take a total of 10 minutes. Try to do it on at least two days a week, morning and evening – or on a daily basis if you wish.

1 Sit comfortably in a chair. Take a few moments to relax and centre yourself. Take some deep breaths and make your exhalations long and smooth. Bring your left foot up on to your right thigh.

2 Using your thumb, gently massage the heart and lung reflexes, which lie between the diaphragm line and the base of your toes. Do this for one minute.

3 Now massage the heart area, which lies between the diaphragm line and the base of your big toe (this area is bigger on the left foot than on the right, because the left ventricle has thicker walls than the right ventricle). Do this for one minute.

4 Massage across the diaphragm line for one minute.

5 Massage along the spinal reflex, which runs along the inner edge of each foot from the top of the big toe to the side of the heel. Do this for one minute.

6 Finally, massage inside the arch of your foot, which contains reflexes relating to your left kidney and adrenal gland. Do this for one minute.

7 Repeat the massage on your right foot.

acupuncture

Acupuncture is part of traditional Chinese medicine (TCM). It is based on the belief that we all have a vibrant life energy, known as qi or chi (pronounced "chee") that flows through the body along specific channels known as meridians. There are 12 major meridians, which correspond to organs in the body. Qi enters the meridians from outside the body, flows in a specific direction along the meridians and nourishes our internal organs in the process.

As long as qi energy flows smoothly along the meridians, we live in a state of health and balance. But if the flow of qi is disrupted by factors such as stress, poor diet and spiritual neglect, there will be an imbalance in energy flow. This results in the symptoms of ill health. According to traditional Chinese medicine, hypertension is believed to result from energy blockages along the liver meridian.

Acupuncture is designed to free energy blockages by the insertion of needles into specific points on

The meridians

There are 12 pairs of meridians in the body. Acupuncture works by stimulating or suppressing the flow of qi energy along these channels at specific places known as acupoints. Blockages in the liver meridian are linked with hypertension.

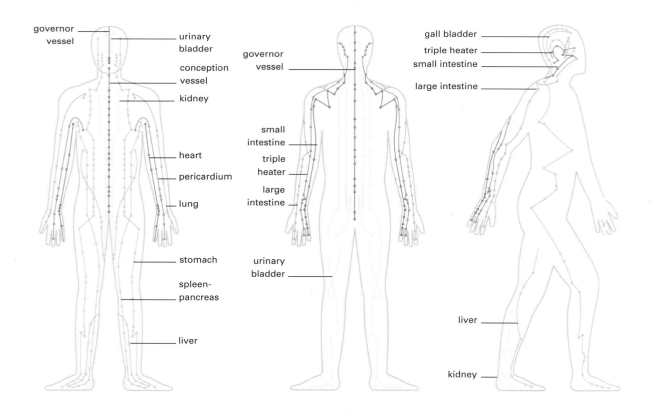

governor vessel
urinary bladder
conception vessel
kidney
heart
pericardium
lung
stomach
spleen-pancreas
liver

governor vessel
small intestine
triple heater
large intestine
urinary bladder

gall bladder
triple heater
small intestine
large intestine
liver
kidney

meridians known as acupoints. An acupoint is a point on a meridian where qi is concentrated and where qi can enter or leave the body.

How effective is acupuncture?

Research suggests that acupuncture can relieve stress by triggering the release of natural, heroin-like chemicals in the brain, and it can lower blood pressure by having an effect on hormone secretion in the body. In a trial published in 1997, 50 people with untreated essential hypertension received acupuncture and, within 30 minutes, their blood pressure fell from an average of 169/107mmHg to 151/96mmHg (with a heart rate reduction from 77 to 72 beats per minute). Blood levels of renin (see page 13), a hormone involved in blood pressure regulation, also fell significantly.

Other studies have shown that acupuncture can improve the function of the left side of the heart, and that it's effective in some people for whom anti-hypertensive drugs have failed. Researchers in California have also shown that acupuncture can blunt the increase in blood pressure that is caused by mental stress – in those receiving acupuncture, blood pressure rose by only 2.9mmHg during periods of stress as opposed to 5.4mmHg in those who were receiving sham acupuncture.

Consulting an acupuncturist

During an initial consultation an acupuncturist will ask detailed questions about your health, emotional state, and your past health and family history. He or she will also assess the flow of qi through your meridians by taking your pulse (there are 12 wrist pulses, six on each wrist, as opposed to the single pulse used in Western medicine) and examine the general appearance, colour and texture of your tongue.

During acupuncture, a therapist stimulates (or sometimes suppresses) the flow of qi by inserting fine, ster-

ile, disposable needles a few millimetres into your skin at selected acupoints. Although you may notice a slight pricking or tingling sensation as a needle is inserted, you should not feel any pain. Needles may be inserted for a few seconds, a few minutes, or up to an hour. They may be flicked or rotated to stimulate qi and draw or disperse energy from an acupoint. In some cases, the action of the needles is enhanced with electricity (called electro-acupuncture) or with a burning herb (called moxibustion). For a long-standing problem such as hypertension, you will benefit from one or two treatments per week for at least two months.

Acupressure

You can stimulate acupoints yourself using finger or thumb pressure. This is known as acupressure and relies on the same underlying principles as acupuncture. Many people are more comfortable with acupressure than with the insertion of needles. You should avoid using acupressure if your blood pressure is 200/100mmHg or higher. However, if your blood pressure is below this, try stimulating suitable acupoints – I suggest one in the box below and two more in the full-strength program on page 160.

> ### Acupressure self-help
> There is an acupoint in Chinese medicine known as LV3 or tai chong ("great surge") that lies on your liver meridian. Stimulating this point helps lower blood pressure by releasing stagnant energy along the liver meridian. To find LV3, place your index finger on the top of your foot, on the web of skin between your big toe and second toe. Then slide your finger 2cm (¾in) along the top of your foot, until you feel a depression between the two underlying bones. Press on this point with your index finger.

yoga

Yoga is an ancient Hindu system of philosophy that uses postures, breath control and meditation to calm the mind and body. Although there are many different types of yoga, all have the ultimate aim of union between your inner self and the divine.

According to yogic theory, the practice of yoga enhances the flow of life-force energy around the body. This energy is known as prana and it flows along channels called nadis (in the same way that qi energy flows through meridians according to the Chinese view of the body; see page 40). When prana flows freely, the body exists in a state of health and balance; when prana is blocked, the body becomes ill.

One of the aims of yoga is to encourage prana to flow up a central channel, or nadi, in the body called sushumna nadi. This channel starts at the base of the body (the perineum) and ends at the crown of the head. Along this channel lie energy centres known as chakras – as energy ascends through each chakra, you experience a different state of consciousness. When energy reaches the crown chakra, you are said to have reached a higher level of consciousness in which you have moved beyond the self – this is the ultimate aim of all types of yoga.

From a Western perspective it's recognized that yoga is a powerful technique for reducing both stress and blood pressure. One study in the medical journal *The Lancet* in 1973 showed that yoga and meditation combined with biofeedback (see page 45) improved hypertension to the point at which 25 percent of participants no longer needed medication, and 35 percent had the doses of their medication reduced. Two years later, another paper in the same journal found that using yoga, relaxation and biofeedback for six weeks could reduce average blood pressure in a group of people with hypertension from an average of 168/100mmHg down to 141/84mmHg.

Starting yoga

Yoga is widely taught in the West. You can find classes in most health and leisure centres, as well as in dedicated yoga centres and retreats. For optimum benefit, yoga should be practised three or four times a week for 30–60 minutes per session. Start slowly, however, in a beginner's class, and gradually increase the amount of time you practise. You can also teach yourself yoga at home. I include some simple yoga poses in Part Three that are beneficial for hypertension.

Types of yoga

When looking for a class, there are various types of yoga to choose from – some are more strenuous than others. Choose a type that matches your fitness level.

Hatha yoga This concentrates on the performance of classical yoga postures and is the most widely practised form of yoga in the West. In a typical class you will be taught poses that flow comfortably from one to another at your own pace. Classes are taught at different levels from beginners to advanced.

Iyengar yoga This is a form of hatha yoga. It uses classical yoga postures with the emphasis on alignment and symmetry within individual postures. In an Iyengar class you will be taught how to use props, such as blocks, to help you get into postures correctly. This

> **Yoga postures to avoid**
> If your hypertension is not fully controlled, avoid inverted postures such as headstands or shoulderstands. Inversion can temporarily increase blood pressure.

!

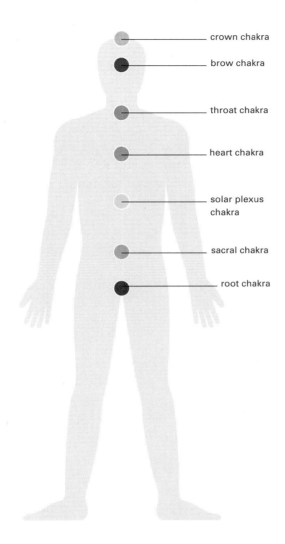

crown chakra

brow chakra

throat chakra

heart chakra

solar plexus chakra

sacral chakra

root chakra

The chakras

Chakras are energy centres that are situated along the midline of your body, from your perineum to the crown of your head. Practising yoga encourages energy to move up through the chakras, bringing physical, emotional and spiritual well-being. Each chakra is associated with particular benefits. For example, meditating on the root chakra, muladhara, releases physical and emotional tension.

form of yoga is ideal for beginners, especially if you are not very fit. I recommend it if you are following the gentle or moderate program (see Part Three).

Viniyoga This is a slow, gentle form of yoga that does not stress your joints. Postures, breath awareness, movements, relaxation, meditation and guided imagery are all used, and are tailored to your individual needs. Viniyoga is ideal if you are unfit, middle-aged or older, or stressed or recovering from illness. I recommend it if you are following the gentle program.

Kripalu yoga This uses meditation and postural alignments to produce a continuous series of spontaneous, dynamic movements. Kripalu yoga is also gentle and relaxing, making it ideal for someone following the gentle or moderate program.

Kundalini yoga This uses postures and breathing exercises along with mantras, meditation, visualization and guided relaxation. It's ideal for those following the moderate program.

Sivananda yoga This uses a series of 12 different poses, relaxation techniques, mantras and breathing exercises. It's ideal for someone flexible who is following the moderate or full-strength program.

Ashtanga yoga This focuses on building strength, suppleness and stamina and is also known as power yoga. Even beginners' classes in ashtanga yoga are fairly strenuous, so this form of yoga is ideal if you are physically fit and following the full-strength program.

Bikram yoga This uses a sequence of yoga postures that are performed in a room heated to at least 38°C (100°F). It's designed to make you sweat profusely and should be avoided if you have hypertension.

qigong

Qigong, pronounced "chee gong", is often referred to as Chinese yoga. It has been practised in China for more than 2,000 years. Qigong is based on the same principle that underlies other Chinese systems of healing such as acupuncture: that life-force energy known as chi or qi flows through channels in the body called meridians. When qi flows smoothly we exist in a state of health and equilibrium, but when its flow is impeded, we become ill. The gentle movements that are characteristic of qigong are designed to regulate the flow of qi through the meridians. "Qi" translates as "energy" and "gong" means "work" or "cultivation".

Research shows that qigong can lower blood pressure (typically by 11/7mmHg) and cholesterol levels, which makes it at least as effective as normal exercise. For people taking anti-hypertensive medication, practising qigong has been shown to reduce the drug dosage required for blood pressure maintenance as well as reducing the incidence of stroke.

Starting qigong

Qigong is usually taught in tai chi classes (qigong movements are often used to warm up before practising the flowing sequence of tai chi movements), but you can also learn qigong from a teacher who practises privately. In the moderate program in Part Three, I provide a series of qigong exercises that are easy to do at home. Even if you don't do the moderate program, you can try the qigong exercises as a taster.

Aspects of qigong

There are many different styles of qigong. Some styles concentrate on static standing postures, others on slow, fluid movements that are similar in appearance to tai chi. Still other styles emphasize meditation. But common to all styles of qigong is the importance that is placed on breathwork and mental focus or visualization. These are considered very important in regulating the flow of qi.

Breathwork When you practise qigong, your breathing should be slow and deep, and penetrate as far as your tan tien (see box below). Allow your movements to fall in time with your breath, rather than the other way round.

Mental focus Visualizing the flow of qi in your body as you practise qigong can greatly enhance the benefits. When you become experienced in qigong, as well as visualizing qi you should be able to feel it flowing in your body – it may manifest itself as a tingling feeling or a warm sensation.

The tan tien

The tan tien is very important in qigong. It is the place inside the body where qi is stored – it's sometimes referred to as the energy powerhouse or reservoir – and it lies 3cm (1¼in) underneath your navel and about one third of the way inside your body in line with the top of your head. At the end of any qigong practice it's important to direct qi back into the tan tien – you do this using your hands, and also by visualizing the flow of qi back into this area. When the tan tien is full of qi, it pumps it in a circuit around the body bringing nourishment and well-being. If you go to classes to learn qigong, you will be taught to breathe deeply into your tan tien. Instead of breathing into your chest cavity, you will be encouraged to draw your breath deep down into your abdomen so your belly expands outward. Over time, this should become your default method of breathing.

meditation

Meditation is a practice that involves focusing the mind to achieve a state of calm and heightened awareness. Those experienced in meditation can quickly enter a trance-like state in which the brain generates special theta waves that are associated with creativity, visions and profound relaxation. Meditation can be practised by itself, but it often goes hand in hand with yoga in helping reduce blood pressure and the adverse effects of stress. At least 20 studies have shown that meditation helps lower blood pressure in people with mild or moderate hypertension.

Starting meditation

You can learn meditation from a teacher or by yourself. I provide some simple meditation exercises that are suitable for everyone in Part Three. Ideally, you should try to meditate for 15–30 minutes for at least five days a week, and preferably every day.

Types of meditation

There are many different ways to meditate and many different traditions, both spiritual and secular, that teach meditation.

Mindfulness meditation This encourages you to focus on your breath to improve awareness of the present moment. You can also practise mindfulness in daily life by focusing on sensations, textures, colours, smells and sounds around you.

Moving meditation This involves quieting your mind through movement such as walking. Movement engages your body and quiets your mind.

Transcendental meditation (TM) This was developed by Maharishi Mahesh Yogi to meet the needs of busy, modern lifestyles – TM is practised twice a day, for 20 minutes each time. TM uses the silent repetition of Sanskrit mantras (short words or phrases) to help you achieve a state of restful alertness. In 2005, a study showed that those practising TM were 23 percent less likely to die from any cause, and 30 percent less likely to die from heart attack or stroke, over an eight-year follow-up period, compared with a similar group of people not practising TM.

Relaxation response meditation This was derived from TM by a Harvard University researcher, Dr Herbert Benson, who wanted to make this form of relaxation more acceptable to Westerners. He took the principles of TM and moved them out of an Eastern context. Instead of Sanskrit mantras, you choose words, such as "relax" or "peace", that are rooted in your own belief system.

Biofeedback and autogenic training

Both biofeedback and autogenic training are therapies that, like meditation, help you lower your blood pressure using the power of your mind. During biofeedback, a practitioner will attach you to devices that monitor your body for sweat production, muscle tension and heart rate (this tells you how stressed or relaxed you are). Information from these devices is constantly fed back to you so you can monitor your level of stress/relaxation as you practise breathing techniques and relaxation exercises. If a particular relaxation exercise works for you, you'll immediately witness a drop in your muscle tension and heart rate. Such feedback provides a direct and powerful way of learning how to relax. Most people learn to lower their blood pressure after just four to six biofeedback sessions.

Autogenic training works on a similar principle to biofeedback but without the monitoring devices. See page 159 for an example of an autogenic training exercise.

nutritional approaches to treatment

A healthy diet can protect against hypertension and other cardiovascular problems by providing vitamins, minerals, antioxidants and other substances (such as phytochemicals) that have a beneficial effect on body function. It's important to avoid eating too much of the wrong sort of food because this can damage your cardiovascular health in the following ways:

- If you are genetically predisposed to hypertension, excess salt may contribute to its development.
- Eating insufficient amounts of fibre increases the absorption of dietary cholesterol and can cause blood cholesterol levels to rise – this can lead to atherosclerosis.
- Eating too much food that contains hydrogenated fat and trans fats (see page 51) increases the risk of atherosclerosis.
- Eating too much carbohydrate raises triglyceride levels and stimulates the secretion of insulin, the main fat-storing hormone in the body. This can lead to weight gain and obesity – a risk factor for atherosclerosis.

- An insufficient amount of antioxidants in your diet contributes to the development of atherosclerosis.
- Insufficient amounts of folate and vitamins B6 and B12 are associated with elevated levels of homo-cysteine (see page 21), which, once again, promote the development of atherosclerosis.

Eating healthily

The guidelines for eating healthily when you have hypertension are based on the results of a series of studies called the Dietary Approaches to Stop Hypertension (DASH) trials. The emphasis in the "DASH diet" is on fruit, vegetables, wholegrains, poultry, fish and low-fat dairy products. The DASH diet recommends cutting down on red meat, saturated fat, cholesterol-rich foods, sodium and sugar. If you follow this diet, you may see significant reductions in blood pressure in just eight weeks. Following the DASH diet not only lowers your blood pressure, it can also increase your levels of "good" cholesterol, lower triglyceride levels and help you lose a significant amount of weight. The following guidelines encompass the principles of the DASH diet. I recommend that you follow them every day.

Eat raw or living foods Where appropriate, try to ensure that half the foods you eat are raw. Processing and cooking destroys antioxidants, vitamins, minerals, enzymes and other phytochemicals, making foods less nutritious. Eat uncooked and unprocessed fruit, vegetables, salad, nuts and seeds. Living foods such as sprouting beans and seeds (for example, alfalfa,

Good diet can protect against hypertension and other cardiovascular problems. Cutting down on red meat, saturated fat, cholesterol-rich foods, sodium and sugar is recommended.

radish, mung bean, broccoli, white radish, red-clover, wheat, lentil, quinoa, and mustard and cress) are high in enzyme and nutrient content because they are still growing. You can find out how to sprout your own beans and seeds on page 111. If you eat raw fish (such as sushi or sashimi) or raw meat (such as steak tartare or carpaccio), ensure it's extremely fresh.

Concentrate on eating fruit and vegetables Aim to eat at least five, and preferably eight to 10 servings of fruit, vegetables and saladstuff per day. Fruit is an exceptionally good source of potassium, antioxidants, fibre and phytochemicals, and has a blood pressure-lowering effect. Apples, avocados, blueberries, cherries, figs, grapefruit, grapes, guava, kiwi, mango and pomegranate (see pages 56–59) are particularly recommended for people with hypertension. Similarly, certain vegetables (broccoli, mushrooms and spinach) and pulses (chickpeas and soybeans) provide benefits for the circulatory system. Salad leaves that are red or dark green provide the most nutrients.

Avoid overcooking vegetables Any form of cooking destroys antioxidants, vitamins and phytochemicals. Boiling, microwaving or frying reduces the carotenoid/ vitamin A content of food by 40 percent after one hour and by 70 percent after two hours (in casseroles, for example). Around 20 percent of folate in vegetables is lost during pressure-cooking and up to 50 percent during boiling and microwaving. Vitamin B2 in vegetables is readily lost into cooking water (it colours the water yellow), and when frozen vegetables are thawed and cooked, 40 percent of vitamin B6 is lost into water. Vitamin C is the most unstable nutrient – up to 50 percent is lost in cooking water when you boil vegetables. Light steaming or brief stir-frying is the best way to preserve nutrients. If you need to boil vegetables, add them to a small amount of boiling water, and cook briefly. Chopping them into coarse chunks rather than thin julienne strips also reduces the surface area over which nutrients are lost. You can reclaim lost nutrients by using cooking water in gravy, sauces and stocks.

Eat healthy fats Eat foods that are rich in omega-3 fatty acids (see page 52), such as oily fish, and certain nuts and seeds. Nuts and seeds are rich not only in healthy fats but also contain magnesium. A handful a day can reduce your risk of a heart attack or stroke. Almonds, Brazil nuts, pumpkin seeds and walnuts (see pages 56–59) and their oils are particularly beneficial.

Eat organic when you can Gram for gram, organic foods consistently provide more nutrients – partly because they tend to contain less water, and partly because they are grown in soils fertilized with natural material rich in trace elements rather than just the potassium, nitrogen and phosphates in artificial fertilizer. Organic foods are also grown for flavour rather than uniformity of size, shape and colour.

Cut back on salt This is one of the most important steps for your cardiovascular health. See my advice on salt intake on page 53.

Select low-glycemic foods These foods cause a slow and steady rise in your blood glucose level (as opposed to high-glycemic foods, which cause a sharp peak; see pages 54–55). Examples of low-glycemic foods include

pulses, wholegrains and brown rice. High-glycemic foods, which should be limited, include sugar, sweet or stodgy foods and potato products – they increase triglyceride levels, trigger the secretion of insulin and can lead to weight gain and glucose intolerance – all of which are bad for cardiovascular health.

Select superfoods As well as fruit, vegetables, nuts and seeds, certain other foods are beneficial for people with hypertension. These include dark chocolate, garlic (and related foods, especially shallots), green tea, oily fish and yogurt (see pages 56–59).

Avoid additives Where possible, avoid foods full of additives such as artificial colourings, flavourings (especially monosodium glutamate), sweeteners (such as aspartame) and preservatives.

Drink plenty of fluid Aim to drink 2–3l (3½–5pt) of fluid per day. Concentrate on drinking water, green tea and unsweetened herbal or fruit teas. Cut back on caffeinated drinks, including coffee, and avoid fizzy drinks (other than water) as these often contain excessive amounts of phosphoric acid, glucose and/or artificial sweeteners, colourings and preservatives.

Take appropriate supplements Although the primary source of nutrients in your diet should be food, nutritional supplements can have a powerful protective effect on your circulatory health (see pages 60–63).

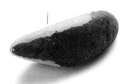 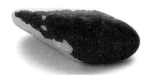 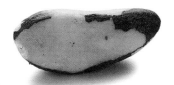 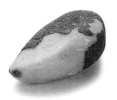

eating more fruit and vegetables

Fruit and vegetables are excellent sources of vitamins, minerals, antioxidants, fibre and plant substances (phytonutrients), all of which have beneficial effects on the circulation. A number of studies show that people with the highest intake of fruit and vegetables have the lowest blood pressure and the lowest risk of developing hypertension, coronary heart disease and stroke.

One study involving 41,541 women with an initially normal blood pressure found that, over a four-year follow-up period, the more fruit and vegetables they ate, the lower their systolic and diastolic blood pressures, regardless of their weight, alcohol and sodium intakes. Apples, oranges, prunes, grapes, carrots, alfalfa, mushrooms, raw spinach, tofu and celery were the fruit and vegetables associated with the most significant reductions in blood pressure.

The power of antioxidants

During normal bodily processes the body produces substances known as free radicals. In excess, free radicals can cause damage to cells throughout the body and lead to the hardening and furring up of the arteries (excess free-radical production may be the result of stress, illness, and exposure to tobacco smoke and pollution, among other things). However, the antioxidants present in fruit and vegetables can neutralize free radicals and prevent the damage they would otherwise do to the body. An antioxidant-rich diet is very important for the health of the heart and blood vessels – a number of studies show that people with hypertension are likely to have low levels of antioxidants.

The main antioxidants in fruit and vegetables are vitamins C and E, beta-carotene (which is converted to the antioxidant vitamin A in the body), and the mineral selenium. But there are also many other equally important antioxidants found in plants. Examples include:

- Polyphenols – found in red grapes, blueberries and cranberries.
- Proanthocyanidins – found in berries and grapes.
- Lycopene – found in tomatoes.
- Quercetin – found in apples, onions and citrus fruit.
- Lutein – found in green leafy vegetables, such as spinach and kale.

Other protective effects

A high intake of fruit and vegetables can protect your cardiovascular system by providing you with an excellent source of the mineral potassium. Your kidneys need potassium to flush excess sodium from your body – this is important because excess sodium is strongly linked to age-related rises in blood pressure.

Fruit and vegetables also provide the B-group vitamin, folate. This is the natural form of synthetic folic acid and it is vital for regulating blood levels of a substance called homocysteine (high levels of homocysteine are linked with cardiovascular disease; see page 21).

In addition, plant hormones called phytoestrogens have a weak, oestrogen-like action on hormone receptors in the circulation. They have been shown to dilate coronary arteries, enhance heart function, reduce blood levels of harmful LDL-cholesterol (see page 51) and reduce blood stickiness. They also possess antioxidant and anti-inflammatory properties. Research consistently shows an association between phytoestrogen-rich diets and a reduced risk of cardiovascular disease.

A high fruit and vegetable intake ensures you get plenty of plant fibre. This helps slow the absorption of dietary carbohydrates and fats, so the level of glucose and fats in your blood remains stable. This in turn reduces your risk of atherosclerosis (see page 15), and therefore hypertension. Plant fibre also encourages a beneficial balance of intestinal bacteria needed to convert phytoestrogens to more powerful forms.

Eating more than five a day

The standard advice is that you should eat at least five servings of fruit and vegetables a day, but you will experience greater benefits if you eat eight to 10 servings a day. Where possible, eat raw fruit and vegetables (or lightly steam them). In particular, "living" foods such as bean sprouts have a high enzyme content. Try the following suggestions:

- Add fruit, such as bananas and grapes, to your breakfast cereal, or stir strawberries or raspberries into yogurt.
- Make salad the basis of your lunch.
- Include several different types of vegetable in your evening meal. Experiment with vegetables you might not have tried before, such as pak choi.
- Where possible, try to replace red meat with vegetables – vegetarians and lacto-vegetarians have lower blood pressure than the general population, regardless of their age, gender and weight.
- Snack on fruit or vegetables (tomatoes, cucumbers or slices of red pepper) when you feel hungry.

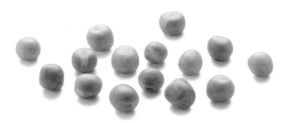

What counts as a serving?

Over a period of time, build up to eating eight to 10 servings of fruit and vegetables a day. Try to make your selection as varied as possible, rather than eating, say, just apples or bananas each day. The following amounts give you an idea of how much fruit or vegetables constitute "a serving". However, another interpretation of a serving is that it's the amount you are happy to eat in one sitting. Generally, the bigger the fruit or vegetable serving, the better. Potatoes do not count toward a vegetable serving as they consist mainly of starch. The same is true of yams. Similarly, don't count vegetables that are canned in salt water, as their benefits are outweighed by the detriments of sodium. Pulses can be counted as a vegetable serving but, unless they are sprouted, they contain little vitamin C. Each of the following measures is equal to one serving:

- A whole apple, orange, pear, peach, nectarine, kiwi, banana, pomegranate or similar sized fruit.
- A couple of satsumas, plums, apricots, figs, tomatoes or similar-sized fruit.
- Half a grapefruit, sweetie, guava, mango, Gaia melon or avocado.
- A handful of grapes, cherries, blueberries, strawberries, dates or other small fruit/berries.
- One tablespoon of dried fruit, such as raisins or cranberries.
- A handful of chopped vegetables/pulses, such as carrots, cabbage, sweetcorn, broccoli florets, beans, peas, lentils or chickpeas.
- A small bowl of loosely packed mixed salad.
- A small bowl of vegetable soup.
- A wine glass (100ml/3½fl oz) of fruit or vegetable juice. This counts toward a maximum of one serving per day, because juice does not contain a significant amount of fibre.

eating good fats

How much fat – and what type – you eat in your daily diet can have a big impact on your long-term health. Some types of fat cause blood levels of unhealthy cholesterol to rise and can lead to clogged and narrowed arteries (or damage them further if you have atherosclerosis). Other types of fat can actually improve the health of your cardiovascular system and reduce your future risk of coronary heart disease.

Unhealthy fats

When hypertension is diagnosed a blood test is carried out to check the levels of certain types of fat in the blood: triglycerides, LDL-cholesterol and HDL-cholesterol (see the box below, and the chart on page 52 for recommended levels of each). Unhealthy levels of these fats exacerbate hypertension and increase the risk of developing cardiovascular problems. Although your family history, and other factors, can affect whether you develop unhealthy levels of blood

Good versus bad cholesterol
Good cholesterol is known as HDL-cho-lesterol (high-density lipoprotein). It's considered good because it transports excess bad cholesterol back to the liver where it can be disposed of. Bad cholesterol is known as LDL-cholesterol (low-density lipoprotein). When it reaches a certain level in your blood, it can start to deposit itself on the inner artery walls, which, over time, blocks your arteries. The ratio of your LDL and HDL levels is important in health terms – if you have high LDL/low HDL, your risk of coronary heart disease increases. You can change this by eating healthily, cutting down on alcohol, exercising and quitting smoking.

fats, your diet plays an important part (and one that is within your control). The following types of dietary fat can increase your risk:

Saturated fats These are fats that tend to be solid at room temperature. They are found in cheese, butter, lard, meat, eggs and palm oil, as well as being present in many processed foods such as cakes, biscuits, pies and pastries. A diet that is high in saturated fat can lead to weight gain and, in some cases, is linked with an increase in the bad type of cholesterol (LDL-cholesterol).

Trans fats These are formed when polyunsaturated oils are partly solidified to make vegetable shortening or margarine in a process called hydrogenation. Trans fats have a molecular structure that hastens the hardening and furring up of the arteries, raises blood levels of bad LDL-cholesterol and lowers levels of good HDL-cholesterol. Trans fats are linked with an increased risk of hypertension and coronary heart disease. Some countries have introduced guidelines aimed at reducing intakes of trans fats to no more than 2 percent of your total energy intake.

Healthy fats

Replacing saturated and trans fats with healthy fats can have a positive impact on your blood fat levels and reduce your chance of health problems.

Polyunsaturated fats These are fats that are liquid at room temperature. They include vegetable oils such as corn oil and sunflower oil. They contain essential fatty acids such as omega-6 and omega-3 fatty acids, both of which are important in the prevention and control of a range of diseases from arthritis to heart disease and cancer. Some polyunsaturated fats lower the levels of bad LDL-cholesterol in your blood. However, too many

Healthy levels of fats in your blood

type of fat	recommended level
Total cholesterol	Below 5 millimoles per litre
Triglycerides	Below 1.7 millimoles per litre
LDL-cholesterol	Below 3 millimoles per litre
HDL-cholesterol	Above 1.2 millimoles per litre

omega-6 fatty acids in your diet can have the opposite effect and cause damage to your body. For this reason, it's advisable to prioritize monounsaturated fats and omega-3s over omega-6 polyunsaturated fats.

Omega-3 fatty acids These are found in polyunsaturated fats but they deserve special mention because they play such an important role in protecting your heart. Omega-3s are found in walnuts, linseeds and linseed oil, and in oily fish such as mackerel, herring, tuna, salmon and trout. Because omega-3s are so important for cardiovascular health, I advise anyone with hypertension to take a fish oil supplement (see my supplement advice in each of the three programs in Part Three).

Monounsaturated fats These are liquid at room temperature, but may solidify at lower temperatures (in the fridge, for example). They include olive oil, rapeseed oil and groundnut oil. Monounsaturated fats are also found in olives, avocados and some nuts (especially macadamias) and seeds. They not only lower your level of bad LDL-cholesterol; they also maintain or even raise the level of good HDL-cholesterol in your blood.

Fats in your day-to-day diet

If you are accustomed to a diet that is high in saturated fat, the eating plans I suggest later on in the book (see Part Three) will ease you into a lower-fat way of eating, with the emphasis on monounsaturated fats such as olive oil, avocados and nuts and seeds. When you go shopping, get into the habit of checking food labels for the fat content of foods (do the same for salt and sugar). Use the following guidelines per 100g (3½oz) or per serving if a serving is less than this:

- 20g ($^7/_{10}$oz) of total fat or more is a lot of fat.
- 3g ($^1/_{10}$oz) of total fat or less is a little fat.
- 5g ($^1/_5$oz) of saturated fat or more is a large amount.
- 1g ($^1/_{25}$oz) of saturated fat or less is a little amount.

In your daily diet use olive or rapeseed oil for cooking, choose low-fat rather than full-fat dairy products, eat meat sparingly and select meat that is low in fat, such as chicken. Eat oily fish and nuts, seeds and avocados for their high monounsaturated fat content.

Healthy nut butters

Everyone is familiar with peanut butter, but did you know that health food shops and on-line stores sell other nut butters, too? These include almond, Brazil nut, macadamia, hazelnut, pistachio and even pumpkin seed butters. Some, especially walnut butter, need refrigeration even before you open them to preserve their nutritional qualities. They are a rich source of monounsaturated fats, protein and antioxidants – especially vitamin E. Buy nut butters that are free from salt, sugar and preservatives (and preferably organic). For a simple lunch, spread some nut butter on a few oatcakes and serve with a light salad and some fruit.

cutting down on salt

We need salt (sodium chloride) for nerve and muscle activity, and to maintain the water balance in the body. The problem is that many of us consume too much of it. Today, the average salt consumption in people following a western diet is between 9g (³/₁₀oz) and 12g (²/₅oz) per day. Yet we evolved on a diet that provided less than 1g (¹/₂₅oz) salt a day, and an average adult weighing 70kg (154lb) can maintain a healthy sodium balance with an intake of as little as 1.25g (¹/₂₅oz) salt per day – as long as he or she does not sweat heavily.

A high salt consumption is a major cause of the age-related rise in blood pressure that is common in the West. Populations with salt intakes of less than 3g (¹/₁₀oz) per day do not have this age-related rise.

How salt causes damage

A high salt diet causes fluid retention, which in turn raises blood pressure. And, in genetically sensitive individuals, consuming too much salt can cause the arteries to stiffen and narrow, and the left ventricle of the heart to thicken so that the heart has to work harder to pump blood. These changes contribute to and exacerbate hypertension.

Researchers estimate that reducing salt intake by 3g (¹/₁₀oz) per day can reduce the incidence of stroke by 13 percent and of coronary heart disease by 10 percent. Reducing salt intake by 6g (¹/₅oz) per day could double this benefit, and reducing salt intake by 9g (³/₁₀oz) per day could potentially triple this benefit.

How to cut down

To cut down on salt, avoid adding table salt to food during cooking, and *never* put a salt cellar on the dining table. Researchers have found that if you stop doing this, blood pressure is reduced by at least 5mmHg. Just this simple step could reduce the incidence of coronary heart disease by 15 percent, and the incidence of stroke by 26 percent within the general population.

Also avoid obviously salty foods such as crisps, bacon or salted nuts; fish or meats that have been cured with salt; and products canned in brine. Even meat pastes, pâtés, stock cubes and yeast extracts have a high salt content and are best avoided.

Adapting to less salt Experiments show that if you are accustomed to highly salted foods, it takes at least one month for salt receptors on your tongue to readjust and start detecting lower salt concentrations. As a result, foods may taste bland during this time. Don't be tempted to add salt – use freshly ground black pepper, garlic, and herbs and spices to add flavour instead. Soon you will start to become more sensitive to the natural flavour in your food. Adding lime juice to food can also help by decreasing the concentration at which your taste buds can detect salt.

Check food labels for salt content

Seventy-five percent of salt is hidden in processed, ready-prepared foods, so it's important to check food labels. A typical microwave meal contains around 5g (¹/₅oz) salt, and a bowl of canned soup has 2g (⁷/₁₀₀oz). Aim to cut down your intake to 3g (¹/₁₀oz) a day or less. If a food label gives salt content as "sodium", simply multiply by 2.5 to obtain the salt (sodium chloride) content. A product containing 0.4g (¹/₁₀₀oz) sodium actually contains 1g (¹/₂₅oz) sodium chloride. A rule of thumb is that, per 100g (3½oz) food (or per serving if a serving is less than this): 0.5g (¹/₅₀oz) sodium per 100g (3½oz) or more is a lot of sodium; 0.1g (¹/₂₅₀oz) sodium per 100g (3½ oz) or less is a little sodium.

following a low-glycemic diet

Foods vary in the effect they have on the level of glucose in your blood – some cause a slow, steady, sustained rise in blood glucose, while others cause fast peaks followed by troughs. Foods in the former category are referred to as "low glycemic", and it's now generally accepted that a low-glycemic diet is good for your long-term health. I also recommend a low-glycemic diet to anyone who wants to lose weight. In contrast, if you eat a lot of high-glycemic foods that make your blood glucose rise quickly, in the long term this can damage your blood vessels and promote the development of atherosclerosis.

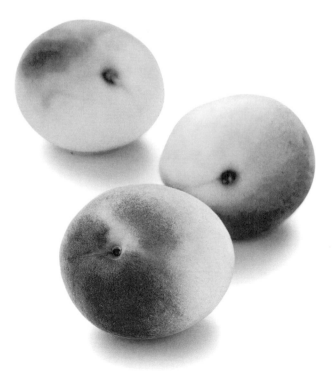

How a food affects your blood glucose depends on how much carbohydrate it contains, and what type. "Complex" carbohydrates, such as brown rice, consist of chains of sugars that are broken down relatively slowly and cause a sustained rise in your blood glucose. "Simple" carbohydrates, found in cakes and confectionery, for example, are rapidly absorbed into your circulation and quickly raise your blood glucose level. Simple carbohydrates are also referred to as simple sugars, and these are the carbohydrate foods I recommend that you avoid or eat in moderation.

What is glycemic index?

In 1981 scientists at the University of Toronto developed the glycemic index (GI) as a way of ranking foods to show how quickly or slowly they cause blood glucose to rise. They gave glucose a rating of 100 (glucose is the simplest type of sugar and is absorbed the most quickly). They then compared how other foods affected blood glucose and rated them accordingly. For example, a food that raised blood glucose levels half as much as glucose was given a GI value of 50. Foods containing lots of simple sugars were given the highest GI rating: 70 or higher. Foods with a low GI, of less than 55, contain carbohydrates that break down more slowly and therefore have only a minor effect on blood glucose levels.

What is glycemic load?

Although GI ratings give us guidance about the effects of different foods on blood glucose, critics point out that GI is not a perfect system. A good way of demonstrating the flaw in the GI system is to look at the example of carrots. They have a middle range GI of 47 yet they would be unlikely to cause a noticeable rise in blood glucose simply because people tend to eat so few of them in one sitting. You would need to eat around two bunches of carrots to produce the blood glucose rise that would be expected from a GI of 47. As a result of the flaws in the GI system, researchers at Harvard University developed the concept of the "glycemic load" (GL), which takes into account the amount of food eaten in a typical serving. The glycemic load is calculated by multiplying a food's glycemic-index value by the amount of carbohydrate found in a typical serving, then dividing the result by 100.

Foods with a GL value of 20 or more are classed as high GL, foods with values of 11–19 are medium GL, and foods with a value of 10 or less are low GL. Using this system, carrots receive a value of three, which means they have a negligible effect on blood glucose and can therefore be eaten in abundance. Books providing GI and GL values are widely available. I have also included some values of common foods in the chart on the right.

Your daily diet

Aim to avoid foods with a high GI/GL and, instead, choose those foods that have a moderate to low ranking. You can also combine foods with a high GI/GL, such as baked potatoes, with those that have a lower GI/GL, such as beans, fish, green vegetables, meat or nuts. This helps prevent fast peaks in your blood glucose levels.

In general, try to cut down on the amount of sugar you eat in your daily diet. Avoid adding sugar to drinks such as tea and coffee, and reduce the amount of sugar you use in home-cooked recipes. Be aware of the amount of sugar in convenience foods; not just soft drinks, cakes and biscuits, but also breakfast cereals and canned products such as baked beans. Get into the habit of checking all the foods you buy for their sugar content. As a guide, when you look at food labels 2g (7/100oz) of sugars or less per 100g (3½oz) is a little sugar, and 10g (2/5oz) of sugars or more per 100g (3½oz) is a lot of sugar.

Glycemic values of some common foods

food	glycemic index value	glycemic load value
parsnips	97	12
baked potato	85	26
wholemeal bread	71	9
fresh pineapple	59	7
wholemeal rye bread	58	8
porridge	58	13
fresh apricots	57	4.9
muesli	56	9
honey	55	10
brown rice	55	18
kiwi fruit	53	6
banana	52	12
unsweetened orange juice	52	12
mango	51	8
new potatoes, boiled	50	14
mixed grain bread	49	6
peas	48	3
carrots	47	3
grapes	46	8
sweet potato	44	11
oranges	42	5
unsweetened apple juice	40	11
apples	38	6
pears	38	4
wholemeal spaghetti	37	16
dried apricots	31	9

superfoods for hypertension

The following foods are considered "superfoods" and I recommend that you include as many as possible in your daily diet. Each one contains valuable nutrients or phytochemicals that have a positive effect on high blood pressure or improve the health of your heart and blood vessels generally. The inclusion of chocolate and wine may surprise you, but evidence suggests that both have a beneficial effect on your cardiovascular system, providing you don't consume too much, and providing you eat dark chocolate and drink red wine.

superfood	cardiovascular benefits	how to use it
almonds Contain vitamin E and antioxidants.	A handful of almonds a day can lower LDL-cholesterol by 4–5 percent and increase HDL-cholesterol by 6 percent. Almond oil has similar benefits. Eating nuts frequently can decrease the risk of coronary heart disease by 30–50 percent.	Eat a handful a day as a snack (about 23 kernels). Or grind to a powder to add to shakes and smoothies, or to sprinkle over cereals and desserts. Use almond oil in salad dressings.
apples One of the richest dietary sources of antioxidant flavonoids, such as quercetin. Despite a relatively high content of fruit sugar, apples have a low GI value, which helps to stabilize blood glucose levels.	Eating an apple a day can reduce the risk of death from any cause at any age (but especially from coronary heart disease or stroke) by one-third, compared with those eating less.	Snack on apples, dried apple rings or apple "crisps". Grate apple flesh and add it to salads and coleslaw (mix it with lemon juice to prevent browning). Use apple in Bircher muesli (see page 100).
avocados Contain mono-unsaturated fat, essential fatty acids and vitamin E. A rich source of potassium. Note: avocados can interact with MAO inhibitors (a type of antidepressant drug) to increase blood pressure.	Daily consumption can increase beneficial HDL-cholesterol by 11 percent within a week. Avocado also boosts your absorption of phytonutrients – if you eat avocado in combination with spinach, your absorption of antioxidant carotenoids is quadrupled.	Use an avocado slicer to remove flesh from the skin easily. Drizzle with walnut or olive oil and eat as a starter. Add avocado flesh to salads. Mix with berries for an interesting fruit salad. Mash to make dips or simply to spread on oatcakes.
blueberries Rich in antioxidants known as anthocyanins and proanthocyanidins.	Daily consumption of 250g (9oz) significantly lowers LDL-cholesterol and blood pressure (by inhibiting the production of angiotensin-converting enzyme; see page 13).	Add a handful of berries to yogurt, muesli, fromage frais, fruit salads or any other dessert. Make your own fresh blueberry juice or smoothie.
Brazil nuts The richest dietary source of antioxidant selenium – a single nut contains around 50mcg. Also a good source of magnesium.	Eating nuts frequently can decrease the risk of coronary heart disease by 30–50 percent.	Eat as a snack, or chop and add to cereal, yogurts and salads. Buy little and often for maximum freshness. Brazil nut butter is a delicious spread.

superfood	cardiovascular benefits	how to use it
broccoli A rich source of folate, phytoestrogens, vitamin C, calcium and magnesium.	The high antioxidant content helps lower blood pressure.	Eat raw, in salads, or lightly steamed or stir-fried.
cherries (black) Provide antioxidant anthocyanins. A good source of vitamin C, plus useful amounts of potassium.	Cherries are thought to have the same health benefits as blueberries.	Eat as a snack, or add to fruit salads and other desserts. Use the flesh when making mixed fruit juices and smoothies.
chickpeas A rich source of antioxidant isoflavones.	Regular intake can reduce total cholesterol and LDL-cholesterol by 4 percent.	Add to soups, stews and salads. Mash to make hummus (see page 141).
chocolate (dark) A rich source of flavonoids – gram for gram, dark chocolate has five times more antioxidant activity than blueberries.	Research found that older men who drank the most cocoa had a blood pressure that was 3.7/2.1mmHg lower than those who drank the least cocoa. They were also half as likely to die of cardiovascular (or any other illness) during a 15-year follow-up.	Eat 40–50g (approx 1½oz) of dark chocolate (at least 70 percent cocoa solids) daily. If you are trying to lose weight, make sure you count the calories in chocolate as part of your daily intake. Drinking unsweetened cocoa is beneficial, too.
coconut Rich in medium-chain fatty acids – these aid the absorption of calcium and magnesium, and are used by the liver as a fuel. Because they are not converted into fat, they increase energy levels and aid weight loss.	Drinking coconut water has been shown to reduce systolic blood pressure by 71 percent and diastolic blood pressure by 29 percent.	Select virgin coconut oil (not odourless, hydrogenated versions) for the greatest health benefits. Use instead of margarine, butter and other oils when cooking and baking. Some experts suggest an intake of 50g (approx 2oz) daily.
figs Rich in polyphenol antioxidants, calcium, potassium and fibre. Gram for gram, dried figs contain more calcium than milk.	Antioxidants prevent oxidation of LDL-cholesterol. The beneficial effect lasts for four hours after consumption.	Eat fresh or dried for an energy-rich snack.
garlic Contains important active ingredients, such as allicin.	Allicin lowers cholesterol levels and blood pressure and makes arteries more elastic.	Eat two or three cloves a day. Add to dishes during cooking. Try the recipe for garlic chicken on page 103.
grapefruit Rich in vitamin C and antioxidants (particularly red grapefruit). See caution on page 83.	One grapefruit a day (either flesh or juice) significantly lowers LDL cholesterol.	Eat as a starter; add to fruit salads; drink freshly squeezed juice.
grapes (red or black) Contain antioxidant anthocyanins and phytochemicals, such as resveratrol, plus potassium and magnesium.	Resveratrol helps lower blood pressure and prevent hardening and furring of the arteries.	Eat a handful of grapes a day or drink a glass of red grape juice. Drinking a glass of red wine daily also provides health benefits.

superfood	cardiovascular benefits	how to use it
green or white tea Contains powerful flavonoid antioxidants such as catechins.	Lowers LDL-cholesterol, blood pressure and blood stickiness. Reduces the risk of heart attack and stroke.	Drink throughout the day. Use left-over cold tea to soak dried fruit. as a base for sauces, soups or stews, or to make ice cream.
guava An excellent source of antioxidant carotenoids, vitamin C, potassium and soluble fibre. Pink guava has an exceptionally high antioxidant content.	Eating several a day for three months has been found to reduce LDL-cholesterol by 10 percent, triglycerides by 8 percent, and blood pressure by 9/8mmHg; and to raise HDL-cholesterol by 8 percent.	Eat for breakfast and add to fruit salads. Drink fresh guava juice or add to smoothies.
kiwi Rich in vitamins C and E, antioxidant polyphenols and potassium.	Eating two or three kiwis a day for 28 days has been found to reduce the potential for abnormal blood clotting by 18 percent, and to lower triglycerides by 15 percent.	Eat with the top cut off, like a boiled egg. Add to fruit and vegetable salads. Include in juices and smoothies.
mango A rich source of antioxidant carotenoids, and vitamins C and E. Also a good source of potassium.	Reduces the constriction of smooth muscle cells in artery walls and may, therefore, reduce stress-related rises in blood pressure.	Eat fresh in fruit salads or on its own. Dried mango makes a deliciously healthy sweet snack.
mushrooms A good source of potassium and selenium. Contain a form of fibre (chitin), plus beta-glutan, which boosts general immunity.	Chitin can lower LDL-cholesterol. Some edible mushrooms, such as *Tricholoma giganteum* (a common species in Japan and Australia), reishi and maitake, can lower blood pressure by blocking angiotensin-converting enzyme (see page 13).	Slice raw into salads; sauté in olive oil with garlic; parboil in bouillon; or bake in the oven, stuffed with mashed butternut squash and parsley. Take reishi or maitake as supplements.
oats A rich source of soluble fibre, beta-glucan and B vitamins.	One bowl of oatmeal a day can reduce LDL-cholesterol by 8–23 percent and reduce blood pressure by 7.5/5.5mmHg over six weeks.	Eat porridge for breakfast; mix rolled oats into yogurt; make home-made unsweetened muesli; and eat oatcakes as a snack.
oily fish A rich source of the omega-3 fatty acids (EPA and DHA), plus vitamins A, D and E.	Eating fish once a week can reduce the risk of a heart attack and stroke.	Eat very fresh fish raw, grilled or baked.
olive oil A rich source of monounsaturated fats such as oleic acid. Extra virgin olive oil, made from the first olive pressing, has the highest antioxidant content.	A diet rich in olive oil reduces the risk of coronary heart disease by 25 percent and the risk of a second heart attack by 56 percent.	Use plain olive oil for cooking. Use extra virgin olive oil in salad dressings and for drizzling on food, and for dipping with bread.

superfood	cardiovascular benefits	how to use it
pomegranate One of the richest dietary sources of polyphenols, anthocyanins and tannins. A good source of vitamins C and E, carotenoids and iron.	Drinking a glass of pomegranate juice a day lowers LDL-cholesterol and can reverse hardening of the arteries. In people with hypertension, drinking 50ml (1⁴/₅fl oz) pomegranate juice twice a day can reduce systolic blood pressure by 5 percent.	Look for fresh pomegranate juice drinks, or make your own. Add pomegranate berries to salads or snack on them.
pumpkin seeds Rich in vitamin E, zinc and a substance called beta-sitosterol.	Beta-sitosterol lowers cholesterol. Eating pumpkin seeds can improve the activity of two groups of anti-hypertensive drugs: calcium channel blockers and ACE inhibitors, producing beneficial therapeutic effects and slowing the progression of hypertension.	Eat a handful as a snack or sprinkle onto salads and cereals. Grind and add to shakes and smoothies.
soybeans A rich source of phytoestrogens (isoflavones).	Evidence shows that consuming 40g (1½oz) soybean protein a day can reduce blood pressure by 7.88/5.27mmHg within 12 weeks in people with hypertension, and by 2.34/1.28mmHg in those without hypertension.	Use soybeans in soups, stews and stir-fries; eat products rich in soybean protein, such as tofu and vegetarian meals (but check salt content first). Add soybean protein powder to smoothies.
spinach One of the richest dietary sources of the carotenoid antioxidants lutein and zeaxanthin.	Substances that inhibit angiotensin-converting enzyme (ACE; see page 24) have been isolated from spinach.	Eat raw or lightly steamed (wilted). Use as an accompaniment to any meal. Baby leaves are great in salads. Try to eat one portion of a dark green leafy vegetable every day.
walnuts Rich in omega-6 and omega-3 fatty acids.	Regular consumption lowers LDL-cholesterol enough to decrease the risk of coronary heart disease by 30–50 percent and increase life span by an estimated 5–10 years.	Add to breakfast cereals, yogurt and salads. Eat as a snack. Use walnut oil as a salad dressing.
wine (red) Rich in antioxidant pigments.	Prevents blood clotting and atherosclerosis; increases levels of HDL-cholesterol.	Drink a glass (150ml/5fl oz) a day.
yogurt Live bio yogurt provides probiotic bacteria, calcium, magnesium and potassium.	Probiotic bacteria can reduce hypertension by blocking angiotensin-converting enzyme (ACE).	Add to cereals and desserts; stir into soups; use in dressings and smoothies. Eat a small carton per day.

supplements for hypertension

The following charts summarize what I feel are the most important supplements for people with hypertension. I explain the role of each supplement, together with the research findings that support its efficacy. I also suggest daily doses. You will find these supplements in my gentle, moderate and full-strength programs in Part Three – there I recommend different dosages for each program.

Many of the following supplements – like the superfoods on the previous pages – are beneficial because they have an antioxidant action in the body. Antioxidants preserve the health of your cardiovascular system and prevent premature aging.

Although a healthy diet should always be the main way to obtain nutrients, food alone often does not supply the quantities of antioxidants, vitamins and minerals needed for optimum protection. Many of the foods we eat in a contemporary Western diet are refined and processed, and this means they have lost many of the vitamins and minerals they started out with.

Supplements are widely available in pharmacies, supermarkets and healthfood stores. They are best taken immediately after food (just four bites of food or a glass of juice will do). If you have not eaten for more than 20 minutes, don't take a supplement. Wait until you have a snack, or drink some juice, and then take it. If taken on an empty stomach, some supplements can make you feel sick or cause indigestion. It's not advisable to take supplements with coffee or tea, as these may interfere with absorption. For tips on how to remember your supplements, see page 82.

When you are taking two or more capsules of the same preparation a day, spread these out over the day, to maximize absorption and obtain more even blood levels of the supplement.

Do not take supplements during pregnancy or breastfeeding except under the advice of a medical herbalist or nutritional therapist. If taking any prescribed medications, check with a pharmacist for any potential supplement-drug interactions.

supplement	research findings	dose and comments
vitamin C An important antioxidant nutrient that combats damage caused by free radicals. A sufficient vitamin C intake also controls the level of the stress hormone cortisol in your bloodstream.	Blood levels of vitamin C have a strong association with systolic blood pressure. People with the lowest blood levels of vitamin C have the highest blood pressure. Research has demonstrated that adding 2g vitamin C daily to an anti-hypertensive drug regime can lower systolic blood pressure by 13mmHg after one month (compared with people who were taking an inactive placebo). The mechanism by which vitamin C lowers blood pressure is not yet understood.	*500–2000mg daily* High doses of vitamin C can result in indigestion. You can avoid this by selecting a supplement described as "non-acidic ester-C". Taking vitamin C supplements can affect laboratory results during some urine or stool tests, so make sure you tell your doctor if you are taking vitamin C.

supplement	research findings	dose and comments

vitamin E An important antioxidant that protects body fats from undergoing damaging oxidation.

Among 2000 people who had previously had a heart attack, those who were given vitamin E supplements for 18 months had a 77 percent lower risk of a further heart attack – in fact, their risk dropped to the level where it was no greater than for people without coronary heart disease. Taking 67mg vitamin E daily for at least two years reduces the risk of coronary heart disease by 40 percent. Centenarians have exceptionally high blood levels of vitamin E, which may contribute to their longevity.

100–600mg daily
Vitamin E is temporarily converted into a free radical as a result of its antioxidant action. For this reason it's important to take it alongside other antioxidants, such as vitamin C, so it's converted back into its antioxidant form.

---

carotenoids These are the yellow-orange-red pigments in plants. Examples of carotenoids include beta-carotene in carrots, lycopene in tomatoes, and lutein in spinach and kale. Carotenoids have an antioxidant action in the body.

A large, international study covering 10 European countries found a significant link between low levels of lycopene levels and increased risk of heart attack. Lycopene-rich tomato extracts can reduce blood pressure by 10/4mmHg within 8 weeks.

Mixed carotenoids: *15mg daily*
Lycopene-rich carotenoids: *15mg daily*
An excess intake of carotenoids can cause yellowness of the skin, but this resolves when the dose is reduced.

---

selenium A mineral essential for the function of five major antioxidant enzymes in the body (known as glutathione peroxidases).

Selenium reduces blood clotting, which protects against coronary heart disease and stroke. Selenium levels are 27 percent lower in people with hypertension, and 30 percent lower in those with coronary heart disease compared with healthy individuals. A five-year study of 1,110 Finnish males (55–74 years) found that a low selenium level almost quadrupled the risk of fatal stroke.

50–200mcg daily
Avoid taking more than the recommended dose of selenium. Excess is toxic.

---

alpha lipoic acid Also known as thioctic acid, this is a powerful antioxidant that is involved in energy production in cells. It regenerates other important antioxidants such as vitamins C and E.

Alpha lipoic acid helps lower blood pressure by reducing the effect of excess sodium on the body (see page 53). Several studies suggest that alpha lipoic acid can reduce oxidative stress and the loss of protein in urine (which may be a sign that hypertension has damaged kidney function). It may therefore protect the kidneys in people with hypertension.

100–600mg daily
Alpha lipoic acid is often combined with l-carnitine (see page 62) in a 1:1 ratio. If you have diabetes, monitor your blood glucose level when you take alpha lipoic acid as it stimulates the uptake of glucose into your muscle cells to lower blood glucose levels.

supplement	research findings	dose and comments
l-carnitine An amino acid needed to regulate fat metabolism in exercising muscles, such as the heart muscle. L-carnitine levels are reduced in people with hypertension.	Helps minimize heart damage in those at risk of a heart attack. Almost a quarter of men taking L-carnitine for four weeks became free of exercise-induced angina. It can also reduce pain on walking in those with hardening of the peripheral arteries.	*100–600mg daily* L-carnitine is often combined with alpha lipoic acid (see page 61) in a 1:1 ratio. Doses of up to 2g daily are well tolerated.
co-enzyme Q10 Improves oxygen uptake and energy production in cells. Acts together with vitamin E. Co-enzyme Q10 is essential if you are taking a statin drug (see page 25), as these switch off co-enzyme Q10 production.	Taking 100mg daily can reduce blood pressure by an average of 10.6/7.7mmHg. One study showed that half of people with hypertension taking 225mg co-enzyme Q10 daily achieved a reduction of at least one (and up to three) anti-hypertensive drugs within four and a half months.	*10–120mg (or more) daily* In some trials people have taken 600mg co-enzyme Q10 daily with no adverse effects. Alpha lipoic acid, L-carnitine and co-enzyme Q10 work synergistically and are often taken together.
bilberry A rich source of anthocyanins – the pigments that give bilberries their blue colour. Also rich in flavonoid glycosides; both have antioxidant and anti-inflammatory actions.	Strengthens and stabilizes blood vessels; reduces permeability of the blood-brain barrier in hypertension; inhibits unwanted blood clotting and reduces the risk of stroke. Especially important for people with hypertension-related eye damage.	*50–500mg daily* Choose a product that is standardized (see page 35) to 25 percent anthocyanins. Take bilberry fruit extracts rather than leaf extracts.
calcium A mineral that plays a vital role in muscle contraction, nerve conduction, blood clotting, energy production and the regulation of metabolic enzymes. The metabolism of calcium is disturbed in hypertension. Taking calcium supplements is advisable for anyone on a low-sodium diet.	Promotes sodium excretion, which helps lower blood pressure. Calcium supplements can reduce average blood pressure over a 24-hour period by 1.9/1.3mmHg. Low intakes of calcium are linked with hypertension and stroke.	*500–1000mg daily* Take a calcium supplement with essential fatty acids if you have a tendency towards kidney stones (but seek medical advice first). Calcium lactate, calcium gluconate, calcium malate and calcium citrate are the most readily absorbed supplements. Bear in mind that, if you are taking a calcium channel blocker drug, the blood pressure-lowering effect of calcium supplements is lost.
magnesium A vital mineral for maintaining the correct salt balance and electrical stability across cell membranes. It is involved in blood pressure control and is especially important in controlling calcium entry into heart cells to trigger a regular heartbeat.	Lack of magnesium increases the risk of developing hypertension and increases the likelihood of spasms in the coronary arteries (linked with angina and heart attack). Magnesium supplements can reduce blood pressure by 2.7/3.4mmHg if you have mild to moderate hypertension.	*300mg daily* Take with food to maximize absorption. Magnesium citrate is most readily absorbed; magnesium gluconate is less likely to cause side-effects such as diarrhea at higher doses. Ensure you have a good calcium intake if you take magnesium.

supplement	research findings	dose and comments
folic acid This is the more easily absorbed, synthetic form of the naturally occurring vitamin folate. Together with vitamin B12, it lowers homocysteine levels (see page 21).	May reduce elevated homocysteine levels by 25 percent. Taking it with vitamin B12 can produce a further 7 percent reduction. Folic acid improves baroreceptor sensitivity (see page 12).	*400–1000mcg daily* Folic acid is usually taken with 50mcg vitamin B12, partly because they work in conjunction with one another, and partly to avoid the masking of B12 deficiency anaemia.
omega-3 fish oil Contains the essential fatty acids: docosahexae-noic acid (DHA) and eicosapentanoic acid (EPA), which are derived from the microalgae on which fish feed. Vitamin E is added to supplements to protect fish oils from oxidation (ran-cidity). Supplementation is important if you are taking a beta-blocker (see page 24), as this drug lowers natural levels of EPA.	Maintains a regular heart rhythm, increases the elasticity of arteries, reduces blood stickiness and reduces blood triglyceride levels by 41 per-cent. Among 11,300 heart attack sur-vivors, those taking supplements had a 15 percent lower risk of heart attack and stroke, and a 30 percent lower risk of cardiovascular death over three and a half years compared with those not taking supplements.	*300–900mg omega-3s daily* (for example, obtained from 1g fish oil capsules, each supplying 180mg EPA + 120mg DHA) Choose emulsified oils to prevent the side-effect of unpleasant belching. Precautions: taking fish oils may affect diabetes control. Seek medical advice if you take a blood-thinning drug such as warfarin.
garlic Provides allicin, a powerful antioxidant.	In people with hypertension garlic can reduce systolic blood pres-sure by an average of 8 percent and diastolic blood pressure by 12 percent within 12 weeks. It also low-ers LDL-cholesterol and triglyceride levels. It reduces blood stickiness, dilates blood vessels and improves blood flow to the peripheral arteries.	*500–1500mg daily* Choose tablets that are stand-ardized (see page 35) to provide 1000–1500mcg allicin. Also choose a product that has an enteric coating – this can reduce the garlic odour on your breath and protect the active ingredients from degradation in the stomach.
reishi mushroom In China this is known as the "mushroom of immortality". Its Latin name is *Ganoderma lucidum.*	Reduces blood clotting, lowers blood pressure and LDL-cholesterol and reduces abnormal blood clotting. Contains substances that lower both diastolic and systolic blood pres-sure in a dose-dependent manner by inhibiting angiotensin-converting enzyme (ACE; see page 24).	*500–1500mg daily* If you are taking immunosuppressive drugs, anticoagulants or cholesterol-lowering medication, you should use reishi only under medical supervision.
probiotics These are live, lactic acid-producing bacteria (for example, *Lactobacillis acidophilus*).	In one study, taking probiotic tablets (12g daily) for four weeks lowered blood pressure by 3.2/5mmHg in people with normal to high blood pressure, and by 11.2/6.5mmHg in those with mild hypertension (compared with people who took an inactive placebo).	Select a supplement that supplies 1–2 billion colony-forming units (CFU) per dose.

lifestyle approaches to treatment

Just about every healthcare professional and complementary therapist will recommend that, alongside your main form of treatment for hypertension, you assess your diet and lifestyle and make changes if you need to. Health guidelines from around the world suggest that you should:

- Keep your caffeine intake within acceptable limits. In particular, minimize your intake of caffeinated drinks such as coffee and cola (see page 65).
- If you smoke, quit – or at least cut down.
- Limit the amount of alcohol you drink to two drinks or fewer per day (see page 67).
- Avoid excessive amounts of stress.
- Introduce rest and relaxation into your life, so that when stress affects you, you can deal with it.
- Take regular exercise – perform 30–45 minutes of aerobic exercise on most days of the week (see page 69).
- Lose weight if you need to. Maintain an ideal body weight with a body mass index (BMI) of between 18.5–24.9 (see pages 70–71).

Collectively, these suggestions are known as lifestyle modifications. Although they may sound simple, in practice they can be among the hardest to achieve. Most people are able to make significant changes to the way they eat, such as increasing their intake of fruit and vegetables and cutting back on salt. Increasing your level of physical activity – and maintaining it – tends to be less simple. And among the most notoriously difficult habits to break are smoking and drinking too much alcohol.

Despite the fact that they pose a challenge, lifestyle modifications are very important – both for people with hypertension and for those at risk of developing it. Changes such as losing weight or quitting smoking can be the most powerful and positive things you do to improve your health and longevity.

If these lifestyle approaches to treatment sound daunting, please don't be put off – my aim in the programs in the next section (see pages 72–173), is to show you how to make sustainable changes in straightforward, enjoyable ways, no matter how fit – or unfit – you are at the moment.

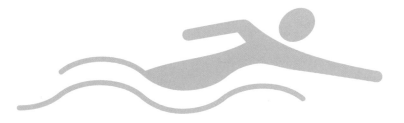

limiting caffeine

Caffeine is a natural stimulant found in some drinks and many over-the-counter drugs, especially those for headaches and colds. The amount of caffeine in a cup of coffee is around 70mg, but can be as high as 150mg if the coffee grounds are brewed for a long time. The average caffeine content of a cup of tea is significantly less: 40mg per cup of black tea; 20mg per cup of green tea; and 15mg per cup of white tea.

The effects of caffeine

Caffeine is a stimulant that mimics the effects of stress hormones: it increases your heart rate, raises your blood pressure and adrenaline levels, reduces your metabolism of glucose and acts on your central nervous system to increase alertness and decrease your perception of effort and fatigue. The extent to which your blood pressure rises in response to a cup of coffee depends on how accustomed you are to caffeine. If you are an infrequent caffeine consumer, two cups of coffee can increase your blood pressure by 5mmHg. If you are a habitual caffeine consumer, individual cups of coffee don't cause the same sudden rise in blood pressure, but this may be because your blood pressure is persistently raised by caffeine anyway.

Everyone metabolizes caffeine at a different rate. The average time taken to metabolize half a given caffeine dose is around four hours, with a range of two to ten hours. Some people metabolize it slowly and get irritable and jittery, while others can drink lots of coffee with no side-effects. The rate at which caffeine is cleared from your system is reduced if you have also been drinking alcohol. A person weighing 70kg (11st) who drinks more than six cups of coffee a day is at risk of caffeine poisoning, with symptoms that can include tremors, nausea, palpitations, anxiety, panic attacks and confusion.

Caffeine is also addictive, in the sense that you become tolerant to it and have to drink more and more to achieve the same stimulant effect. If you stop a high intake of caffeine suddenly, you may have withdrawal symptoms such as headaches, fatigue, sweating, anxiety and muscle pains – these typically last for around 36 hours.

Cutting down on caffeine

If you have hypertension, it's worth minimizing your caffeine intake. If you drink many cups of coffee or a lot of cola every day, cut down by one caffeinated drink a day to avoid withdrawal symptoms. Try to switch slowly to decaffeinated brands and make coffee less strong by brewing grounds for a shorter length of time, or by using fewer instant granules.

Alternatively, try switching to green or white tea. This provides a lower level of caffeine plus beneficial antioxidants. The benefits of tea drinking outweigh the adverse effects of caffeine – evidence suggests tea can protect against coronary heart disease. Herbal teas such as rooibos are also good – rooibos is made from a South African shrub and is high in antioxidants.

How caffeine affects you
Try this simple test to assess the effects of caffeine on your blood pressure. Make your usual cup of coffee but, rather than drinking it straight away, wait for 10 minutes. Spend this time reading a book or listening to music – or doing any activity that will help you to relax. Now check your resting blood pressure using a home monitoring device (see page 22). Drink your coffee and check your blood pressure at 10-minute intervals for the next hour to see whether or not your caffeine intake affects your blood pressure.

quitting smoking

Smoking reduces the amount of oxygen in your blood; it makes your blood more sticky and prone to clotting; and it damages your arteries. In the long term it increases your risk of hypertension by at least 30 percent and your risk of coronary heart disease seven-fold. It also quadruples your risk of having a stroke.

The effects of smoking

Every time you smoke a cigarette, your blood pressure can rise by 9/8mmHg. If you both smoke a cigarette and drink coffee, the increase is even greater and, in some people, is as high as 21/17mmHg. (Nicotine replacement products are therefore not a good idea to help you quit smoking if you have uncontrolled hypertension.)

In the long term, chemicals in cigarette smoke damage the linings of your artery walls, causing inflammation that hastens the hardening and furring up of the arteries (and makes hypertension worse). Long-term smokers tend to have thicker, less elastic arteries, and enlargement of the left ventricle of the heart. Smoking has also been shown to increase the risk of poor kidney function. In addition, people who smoke

Watch your weight
When you quit smoking make sure you don't experience a subsequent increase in your weight and waist measurements – this may offset the expected decrease in your risk of coronary heart disease and stroke. See pages 70–71 for advice about achieving and maintaining a healthy weight.

and have hypertension tend to require more drugs to control their hypertension. This is because smoking reduces the effectiveness of anti-hypertensive drugs, especially beta-blockers and angiotensin II blockers.

If you smoke, consider taking pycnogenol – extracts from the bark of the French maritime pine. A dose of 125mg pycnogenol is as effective in preventing susceptibility to blood clots in smokers as 500mg aspirin, but without the stomach irritation that aspirin causes.

Stopping smoking

The benefits of stopping smoking are soon realized. Within eight hours, levels of oxygen in your circulation increase; within 48 hours, the stickiness of your blood reduces, and within three months your peripheral circulation significantly improves.

Find support to help you quit – stopping smoking is easier if you do it with a friend or relative. Focus on getting through each day – try not to think long term, as this can be daunting. Keep your hands busy with activities such as drawing, painting, origami, knitting, embroidery or DIY – psychologists have found that the hand-to-mouth habit is one of the things that makes quitting smoking so difficult. Increasing the amount of exercise you take will help to curb withdrawal symptoms by increasing secretion of opium-like endorphins. It's also important to identify situations in which you used to smoke, and either avoid them or plan coping strategies in advance. For example, you could practise saying: "No thanks, I've stopped" or "No thanks, I'm cutting down."

To help overcome nicotine cravings, try sucking on an artificial cigarette or herbal stick; do 30 minutes of brisk exercise; take a flower remedy (such as rescue remedy) or try essential oil products designed to reduce cravings. All these aids are available from pharmacies. If you do use nicotine replacement products to help you quit, monitor your blood pressure closely.

limiting alcohol

In small quantities alcohol has a beneficial effect on blood pressure in that it acts as a diuretic and increases sodium loss. Alcohol also increases levels of beneficial HDL-cholesterol and lowers harmful LDL-cholesterol (see page 51). Red wine is particularly beneficial for people with hypertension because it's rich in antioxidants and offers protection against coronary heart disease. As a result, drinking up to 150ml (5fl oz) red wine a day is recommended – you'll notice that I include a glass of red wine in the eating plans in Part Three. If you prefer not to drink alcohol, unsweetened red grape juice provides the same antioxidant benefits, thanks to the phytochemicals present in the grapes.

Adverse effects of alcohol

If you have three or more drinks a day, the benefits of alcohol start to reverse. A high alcohol intake leads to sodium retention, and increases your resistance to the hormone insulin, both of which contribute to hypertension. Above an intake of three drinks (30g/1oz alcohol) per day, every additional drink (10g/⅓oz alcohol) increases your average systolic blood pressure by 1–2mmHg, and diastolic blood pressure by 1mmHg. Excess alcohol also affects your heart (leading to irregular heart rhythms and cardiac enlargement) and your liver (leading to fibrosis and cirrhosis). Excessive alcohol intake is most harmful when it occurs without food. Women are more susceptible to the adverse effects of excessive alcohol than men. Even if you haven't had an alcoholic drink for several days, avoid binge drinking.

If you are overweight (see pages 70–71), you need to monitor your alcohol intake carefully. Being overweight or obese can worsen hypertension and increase your risk of cardiovascular problems. Alcohol is a source of extra calories in your diet – a glass of dry white or red wine contains around 90 calories (sweet white wine contains more), as does a glass (275ml/9⅔fl oz) of beer. A pub measure of spirits (25ml/9/10fl oz) such as whisky, gin or vodka contains around 50 calories, and significantly more if you mix it with a sugary mixer such as cola, lemonade or tonic.

Reducing your alcohol intake

If you drink more than 20g/⅔oz alcohol per day, aim to cut down. Each drink you forgo will lower both your systolic and diastolic blood pressure by around 1mmHg. To work out your daily alcohol consumption, 10g/⅓oz alcohol is equivalent to:

- 300ml (½pt) beer
- 100ml (3½fl oz) wine
- 50ml (1¾fl oz) sherry
- 25 ml (9/10fl oz) spirits

If you are a very heavy drinker, ask your doctor to help you start drinking less – stopping abruptly can cause your blood pressure to rise. If you are a light to moderate drinker, try the following suggestions:

- Put your glass down between sips.
- Savour each sip, holding it longer in your mouth.
- Alternate alcoholic and non-alcoholic drinks.
- Choose unsweetened fruit juices or non-alcoholic cocktails, such as mango juice with coconut milk.
- Try sparkling mineral water with lime juice.
- Try tonic water with a dash of Angostura bitters instead of a gin and tonic.
- Mix chilled wine with sparkling mineral water for a refreshing spritzer.
- Elderflower cordial diluted with mineral water makes a great substitute for white wine.
- A herb known as kudzu (Japanese arrowroot), reduces alcohol cravings. Research suggests this action is due to substances known as isoflavones.

overcoming stress

When you feel stressed, your body prepares for activity as part of its ancient flight or fight response. Nerve signals from your brain trigger the release of adrenaline (epinephrine), noradrenaline (norepinephrine) and cortisol from your adrenal glands, all of which increase blood pressure by constricting peripheral arteries. For ancient humans, this ensured more blood went to the muscles and brain (for fighting and fleeing), and it minimized blood loss as a result of wounds. After the battle was fought (or ancient humans had run away), blood pressure returned to normal.

In modern life, however, stress rarely results in fighting or fleeing, and the affects of adrenaline, noradrenaline and cortisol can persist in the circulation over prolonged periods of time. In susceptible individuals this results in overactivity of the sympathetic nervous system as part of the stress response. Instead of short-lived rises in blood pressure, stress causes blood pressure to become persistently raised.

Combating stress

I would advise everyone, with or without hypertension, to take steps to reduce their exposure to stress or to find strategies for dealing with it. Here are some suggestions that everyone can try:

- Stop what you are doing and inwardly say "calm" to yourself. Combine this with the following step.
- Take a deep breath in and let it out slowly, concentrating on the movement of your diaphragm. Do this two or three times until you feel more in control.
- If you are sitting down, stand up and gently stretch to your fullest possible extent. Shake your hands and arms briskly, then shrug your shoulders.

- Go for a brisk walk, even if it's only briefly around the room. Regular brisk, non-competitive exercise is one of the best ways to lower stress hormones.
- Go somewhere private and groan or shout as loudly as you want. Some people find it helpful to punch a soft cushion as hard as possible.
- Place a few drops of a flower essence such as rescue remedy under your tongue.
- Listen to calming background music – natural sounds like recordings of the sea, bird songs, a babbling brook or a waterfall are ideal.
- Organize your life, make comprehensive lists and manage your time more effectively – prioritize tasks so you can deal with pressures one at a time. Where possible, try to delegate to others.
- Say "no" to unreasonable demands.
- Make a point of complimenting those around you – making others feel good will make you feel good.
- Watch a comedy or do something that makes you laugh – laughter is a great antidote to stress.
- Use visualization or meditation to find calm.

Gaisbock's syndrome
Stress is now linked with a condition known as Gaisbock's syndrome, in which blood pressure goes up and down significantly over relatively short periods of time during the day. Gaisbock's syndrome is a strong predictor of future hypertension. It's also associated with poor function of the left ventricle of the heart and decreased elasticity and increased stiffness of the artery walls. Gaisbock's syndrome is thought to be the cause of white-coat hypertension, in which blood pressure suddenly becomes high when measured (usually by someone wearing a white coat) in a stressful situation, such as a doctor's surgery or hospital (see page 20).

taking regular exercise

We now know that regular aerobic exercise has profound benefits for the cardiovascular system. Among other things, it lowers raised blood pressure and reduces the risk of premature death from coronary heart disease by more than 40 percent.

How much exercise?

Studies suggest that it's wise to exercise every day. Physical activity doesn't need to be intense. Brisk walking for 30–60 minutes a day, most days of the week, produces significant benefits for people with hypertension. In fact, activities such as DIY, gardening and dancing – anything that leaves you feeling warm and slightly out of breath – are as effective as swimming or cycling for cardiovascular health. Yoga and qigong (see pages 42–44) are good for bringing balance, equilibrium and relaxation.

Researchers have found that aerobic exercise doesn't have to take place in a single session – two or three daily sessions of 10–15 minutes are just as good.

Exercising at the right intensity

Try to exercise briskly enough to raise your pulse above 100 beats per minute, raise a light sweat and make you slightly breathless – but not so briskly that you cannot hold a conversation.

Measuring your pulse rate during exercise will ensure that you stay within the safe range for burning excess fat and improving cardiovascular fitness without over-stressing your heart.

Take your 10-second pulse every 10 minutes or so as you exercise. Simply look at your watch and count the number of pulses you feel during a 10-second period. Your pulse is most easily felt on the inner side

10-second pulse ranges	
age group	pulse range
20–29	20–27
30–39	19–25
40–49	18–23
50–59	17–22
60–69	16–21
70+	15–20

of your wrist on the same side as your thumb or on the side of your neck, just under your jaw.

If you are unfit, make sure your pulse stays at the lower end of your 10-second pulse range at first, then slowly work up to the upper end over several weeks. Consult the chart above to find the recommended 10-second pulse range for your age.

If at any time your pulse rate goes higher than it should, stop exercising and walk around slowly until your pulse falls. At the end of 20 minutes' exercise, you should feel invigorated rather than exhausted.

Exercising safely

Warm up and cool down before and after any form of exercise with a few simple bends and stretches. This helps to avoid muscle injuries, and pain and stiffness. For comfort, wear loose clothing and footwear specifically designed for the exercise you have chosen. Don't exercise straight after a heavy meal, after drinking alcohol or if you feel unwell. Stop exercising immediately if you feel very short of breath or unwell. If you are taking medication, seek medical advice before starting an exercise program.

maintaining a healthy weight

If you have hypertension, losing a relatively small amount of excess fat will significantly lower your blood pressure. If you combine exercise with losing weight, the blood pressure-lowering effect is even greater.

Assessing your weight

Your weight is usually assessed using the body mass index (BMI), but another factor to take into account is *where* you store fat – on your hips or on your waist. Fat deposits on your waist are associated with an increased risk of cardiovascular problems.

Body mass index According to the World Health Organization, if your BMI is 18.5 or under, you are underweight; if it's between 18.5–24.9 your weight is ideal; if it's between 25–29.9, you are overweight; and if it's 30 or above, you are obese. Calculate your BMI using the formula described below. (Please note that BMI values are less accurate if you are very muscly or frail – ask your doctor). You can also assess whether you are a healthy weight by consulting the weight ranges in the chart on the opposite page.

Waist size If you store excess fat around your waist in an apple-shape, you are twice as likely to develop hypertension and coronary heart disease as someone who is pear-shaped, with excess fat around their hips.

Having a waist size between 80–88cm (32–35in) for women, or 94–102cm (37–40in) for men, carries a similar health risk as a BMI of 25–30 – it means you are overweight and increases your risk of heart disease by a factor of 1.5. Women with a waist circumference larger than 88cm (35in) and men with a waist circumference larger than 102cm (40in) have an even greater risk of heart disease.

Waist size reductions of just 5–10cm (2–4in) can significantly lower your blood pressure and reduce your risk of a future heart attack.

Calculating BMI

You need two measurements: your weight in kilograms and your height in metres. For example, 76kg and 1.7m

Calculate your height squared. For example: 1.7 x 1.7 = 2.9

Divide your weight by your squared height. For example, 76/2.9 = 26.2. This gives you your BMI, which allows you to assess how healthy your weight is.

Losing excess weight

If you are overweight, try to lose weight slowly and steadily until you reach the healthy range for your height. If you manage this, you should notice significant reductions in your blood pressure and, if you are on anti-hypertensive medication, your doctor may be able to reduce the dose and/or number of anti-hypertensive drugs you are taking.

The best way to lose weight permanently is controversial. In the past, healthy eating messages have consistently recommended low-fat diets to reduce the incidence of obesity and coronary heart disease. Unfortunately, research shows that low-fat diets can lower the level of healthy HDL-cholesterol and increase the level of unhealthy LDL-cholesterol in your body, which may in turn increase the risk of coronary heart disease.

In contrast, a number of studies suggest that following a low-carbohydrate diet can promote weight loss, lower hypertension by 1–10mmHg and reduce LDL-cholesterol and triglycerides while raising HDL-cholesterol and improving blood glucose control.

Extremely low carbohydrate diets such as the Atkins diet do not suit everyone. In my opinion, the ideal compromise appears to be a low-glycemic diet, in which carbohydrates that produce rapid increases in blood glucose levels are avoided (see pages 54–55). This makes sense, as carbohydrates increase the secretion of insulin – the main fat-storing hormone in the body. Most people with hypertension will benefit from cutting back on carbohydrates, especially if they also tend to store fat around the waist.

When you follow my eating plans in the programs in the next part of the book, you should be able to lose weight slowly over a period of weeks and months. This means that instead of dieting to achieve weight loss, you adopt new, healthier eating habits – ones that you will be able to sustain in the long term and ones that will enable you to keep weight off permanently.

The healthy weight for your height

metres/feet	kilograms	stones
1.47/4'10"	40–53.8	6st 4lb–8st 6lb
1.5/4'11"	41.6–56	6st 8lb–8st 11lb
1.52/5ft	42.7–57.5	6st 10lb–9st
1.55/5'1"	44.4–59.8	7st–9st 5lb
1.57/5'2"	45.6–61.4	7st 2lb–9st 9lb
1.6/5'3"	47.4–63.7	7st 6lb–10st
1.63/5'4"	49.2–66.2	7st 10lb–10st 5lb
1.65/5'5"	50.4–66.6	7st 13lb–10st 7lb
1.68/5'6"	52.2–70.3	8st 3lb–11st
1.7/5'7"	53.5–72	8st 6lb–11st 4lb
1.73/5'8"	55.4–74.5	8st 10lb–11st 10lb
1.75/5'9"	56.7–76.3	8st 13lb–12st
1.78/5'10"	58.6–78.9	9st 3lb–12st 5lb
1.8/5'11"	60–80.7	9st 6lb–12st 9lb
1.83/6'	62–83.4	9st 10lb–13st 1lb
1.85/6'1"	63.3–85.2	9st 13lb–13st 5lb
1.88/6'2"	65.4–88	10st 4lb–13st 11lb
1.9/6'3"	66.8–89.9	10st 7lb–14st 1lb
1.93/6'4"	68.9–92.8	10st 12lb–14st 8lb

The natural health guru programs

Having explained what high blood pressure is in Part One, and how it can be treated naturally in Part Two, Part Three offers you the **tools to transform your life**. First, I ask you to complete a questionnaire (see pages 75–76). Your answers will help to identify the best program for you as an individual: the gentle, moderate or full-strength program. **The gentle program** is aimed at people who know they have diet and lifestyle issues to address. It offers you an eating plan that supplies nutritious foods that will benefit your health. **The moderate program** is aimed at people who want to enhance an already healthy diet and lifestyle. **The full-strength program** incorporates all the superfoods that research suggests have the most powerful effect on hypertension – this program is designed to achieve the greatest result in the shortest time. Each program supplies **daily menu plans**, healthy salt-free recipes, **daily exercise routines** and suggestions for therapies to try at home. The programs last 14 days but they can be repeated so they last for 28 days in total. Once you have followed a program, you should notice **significant changes in your blood pressure** and well-being. You can then choose to continue with the diet and lifestyle principles outlined in your program, or you can move on to the next program.

the natural health guru questionnaire

Before you start on the programs in this section of the book, I'd like you to answer the questions on the next two pages. Your answers will give you an overview of your current health, diet and lifestyle habits and help you to decide which is the best program to start with. Whereas a fit 35-year-old with borderline hypertension may be able to start on the full-strength program, an overweight 70-year-old on several medications for hypertension would be better off with the gentle program, at least at first. Age isn't always an indicator of health and fitness, however. A very overweight 30-year-old, who rarely exercises and eats lots of takeaways should start with the gentle program, despite his age. Likewise, a slim, fit grandmother of 70 years, with an adventurous approach to life may be able to start on the moderate program.

Answer A, B or C to each of the 30 questions – whichever seems the closest to your ideal response. If you answer:

- Mostly As: it's a good idea to start with the gentle program.
- Mostly Bs: you may wish to start on the moderate program.
- Mostly Cs: you can follow the full-strength program.

All three programs are based on the principles of the DASH diet (see page 46) and encourage you to eat plenty of fruit and vegetables and wholegrains, and cut down your intake of salt, sugar and unhealthy fats. The gentle program consists of foods that will be familiar to you and includes a small amount of red meat. In the moderate and full-strength programs, I encourage you to adopt an increasingly vegetarian or fish-based diet, and to eat more of the superfoods that are beneficial for hypertension. I also suggest sprouting your own beans and seeds and making your own fruit and vegetable juices in the moderate and full-strength programs. The amount of exercise I recommend in the programs varies from 15–20 minutes in the gentle program to 30–45 minutes in the full-strength program.

Please note that although it may be tempting to start on the full-strength program straight away (because it provides the most benefits), it's unwise to do this if you answer mostly As. It is more beneficial to begin gently and build up over time so that your body becomes accustomed to the changes in your diet and activity levels.

Another way of tackling the programs is to do each one in turn, regardless of your current health and lifestyle: if you opt for this approach, begin with the gentle program, then work your way up to the moderate and the full-strength program. This provides you with three months of menu plans and exercise routines.

If you are taking any prescribed medications, or if you are pregnant, or planning to be, seek medical advice from your doctor before embarking on major dietary and lifestyle changes. If you have diabetes (Type 2 diabetes and hypertension are often associated), you will need to monitor your blood glucose closely as you change your diet and activity levels.

1 How old are you?
A 50 years or older
B 30–50 years
C 30 years or under

2 Do you have hypertension?
A Yes
B Borderline hypertension
C No, but it runs in my family

3 Are you currently taking medication for hypertension?
A Yes, I'm taking more than one anti-hypertensive drug
B Yes, I'm on one anti-hypertensive drug
C No

4 Are you overweight?
A Yes, I need to lose at least 6.4kg (1st)
B Yes, I need to lose less than 6.4kg (1st)
C No, I'm in the healthy weight range for my height

5 Do you tend to store fat around your waist and tummy rather than your hips?
A Yes, I'm apple-shaped
B No, I'm pear shaped
C No, but beer bellies run in my family

6 Do you have diabetes?
A Yes
B No, but diabetes runs in my family
C No, and I have no family history of diabetes

7 Do you have high cholesterol levels?
A Yes
B No, but cholesterol problems run in my family
C No

8 Have you ever had a heart attack?
A Yes
B No, but heart attacks run in my family
C No, and I have no family history of heart attacks

9 Have you ever had a stroke?
A Yes
B No, but strokes run in my family
C No, and I have no family history of strokes

10 What is your resting heart rate? (Skip this question if you are taking a beta-blocker drug.)
A 80 beats per minute or more
B 70–80 beats per minute
C Fewer than 70 beats per minute

11 Do you smoke cigarettes?
A Yes (but I'm trying to quit)
B I used to, but quit in the past five years
C No

12 How much alcohol do you drink?
A Women: more than 14 units per week
Men: more than 21 units per week
B Women: 14 units per week or fewer
Men: 21 units per week or fewer
C None or very little

13 How many caffeinated drinks, such as coffee or cola, do you drink a day?
A More than six
B Between three and six
C Two or less

14 Do you regularly feel you are under a lot of stress?
A Yes, all the time
B Yes, once or twice a week
C No, I'm quite laid back

15 Do you regularly feel anxious or panicky?
A Yes, virtually all the time
B Yes, several times a week
C No, only occasionally

16 How often do you experience headaches?
A Several times a week
B Occasionally
C Hardly ever

17 Do you feel that you lack energy or are exhausted?
  A Yes, regularly
  B Occasionally
  C No, not at all

18 How often do you exercise (or have a high level of physical activity; for example, gardening)?
  A I have not yet managed to fit regular exercise into my life
  B I exercise for 30 minutes two or three times a week
  C I exercise for at least 30 minutes on at least five days a week

19 Are you a vegetarian?
  A No
  B No, but I regularly have days in which I don't eat meat
  C Yes

20 On how many days of the week do you eat meat?
  A Every day or most days
  B Several days
  C One day or less

21 How often do you eat processed and pre-packaged foods?
  A Most days
  B Several times a week
  C I rarely/never touch them

22 How often do you eat takeaways?
  A Several times a week
  B Around once a week
  C I rarely/never touch them

23 How often do you eat fried foods?
  A Several times a week
  B Around once a week
  C I rarely/never touch them

24 Do you eat at least five portions of fruit/vegetables a day?
  A No, I eat fewer than five
  B Yes, I eat at least five
  C Yes, I usually eat more than five

25 How often do you eat fish?
  A Hardly ever
  B At least once or twice a week
  C Three or more times a week, or I take a daily fish oil supplement

26 How often do you add salt to your food?
  A I always add salt during cooking, and add salt to my food at the table
  B I've stopped adding salt during cooking, but sometimes add it at the table
  C I do not add any salt to my food, and I check labels for sodium content

27 Do you follow a low-fat diet?
  A Not really
  B Yes, I've switched to low-fat products (for example, milk)
  C Yes, I always check labels for fat content

28 Do you eat a low-sugar diet?
  A Not really
  B Yes, I've cut right back on sweets and snacks
  C Yes, I always check labels for sugar content

29 Would you describe yourself as an adventurous eater?
  A No, not at all
  B I try to eat at least one new dish each week
  C Yes, definitely

30 Are you willing to change the way you eat significantly?
  A I'll start gently and see how I go
  B Yes, I want to make a difference without going wild
  C Yes, whatever it takes

starting the programs

Now you have decided which program is right for you, you can set a date on which to start. Rather than aim for an immediate start, give yourself a few days to read through the program and gather the things you need. You will need to go food shopping and buy items such as essential oils and supplements, as well as booking appointments with complementary therapists (I recommend visits to two therapists per program).

It's a good idea to create a profile of your current health status before you begin the program (see the chart below). Make a copy of the chart and fill in your statistics at the beginning and end of each program. This will give you a clear idea of what improvements you have made. Seeing the benefits presented in a tangible way can act as a powerful motivator to continue with the diet and lifestyle changes you have made.

Although you can go to your doctor or a pharmacist for a blood pressure reading, I strongly advise you to invest in a home blood pressure monitoring device if you haven't already. Those that automatically inflate around your wrist are the easiest to use. Before you start a program, measure your blood pressure regularly throughout the day for a couple of days – calculate the average reading and enter this in the chart below.

As well as weight and blood pressure, I have also allowed space for you to enter your cholesterol, triglyceride and homocysteine (see pages 21, 51) levels at the beginning and end of a program. If you can have these measured, I recommend that you do. The levels of fats and homocysteine in your blood are a strong indicator of how healthy your cardiovascular system is – and how likely you are to develop coronary heart disease. If your levels decrease, as I would expect, this really helps to underline how much your dietary and lifestyle changes are improving your health. Your doctor should be happy to arrange these tests for you. They are also available from private health screening organizations and many pharmacies.

Progress chart for the gentle, moderate and full-strength programs

measurement	start date	finish date	improvement
Weight			minus
Blood pressure			minus
Total cholesterol			minus
LDL-cholesterol			minus
HDL-cholesterol			plus
Triglycerides			minus
Homocysteine			minus

introducing the gentle program

The gentle program aims to ease you into diet, exercise and lifestyle changes as painlessly as possible. It provides 14 daily plans that you can repeat to create a program lasting for 28 days. It may take a while to settle into the program but, once you get accustomed to the diet and lifestyle changes, feel free to make your own adjustments that take into account your personal likes, dislikes and lifestyle.

The gentle program diet

The daily food plans in the gentle program should not be radically different from your current way of eating. They are designed to introduce you to a lower glycemic index (GI) diet (see pages 54–55) with less refined carbohydrate than you may be used to. The diet also follows the principles of the Dietary Approaches to Stop Hypertension (DASH; see page 46), in which the emphasis is on fruit, vegetables, saladstuff, nuts, wholegrains, poultry, fish and low-fat dairy products.

This approach increases your intake of fibre, antioxidants (especially carotenoids), vitamins (including folate), minerals (such as potassium, magnesium and calcium), and monounsaturated and omega-3 fats. It reduces your intake of sodium, saturated fat, trans fats and cholesterol. Research suggests that this has the potential to lower your blood pressure by 4/2–7/4mmHg or more within 30 days, even if you are taking anti-hypertensive medications (various trials show that DASH enhances the effects of prescribed drugs).

In addition to lowering blood pressure, the gentle program diet may also lower your total and LDL-cholesterol and your triglyceride levels. People who are older, and those who previously had high intakes of salt (sodium chloride) are likely to experience the greatest benefits from the gentle program.

If you wish, you can have one 150ml (5fl oz) glass of red wine per day during the gentle program. Research shows that a daily glass of red wine can reduce the risk of coronary heart disease by one third. If you prefer to avoid alcohol, you can have a glass of unsweetened red grape juice instead. This provides the same heart-healthy antioxidants as red wine, and research suggests that grape juice is at least as good as red wine in improving dilation of arteries. It does not have the same beneficial effect on cholesterol levels, however. You may also include a daily 40–50g (approx 1½oz) piece of dark chocolate (at least 70 percent cocoa solids) during the gentle program.

Foods to avoid or eat less of While on the gentle program it's important to avoid refined carbohydrates (for example, cakes, biscuits and sugary drinks), processed foods (for example, tinned meat and packet soups), sweets and excess alcohol. These foods make hypertension worse – eliminating them and following a healthy eating plan can bring your blood pressure down quite significantly in a relatively short amount of time.

Begin the program by looking at the food labels of any tins, packets and jars in your kitchen cupboards. Throw away all foods containing a lot of saturated fat, sodium or salt, or sugar. For guidelines about what constitutes a "lot" of these ingredients, see pages 52,

Shopping list

These are items that I suggest you buy on a regular basis. They are featured in the suggested meals for the next 14 days. Where possible, buy regularly in small quantities for freshness.

drinks
almond and soy milk, black, green or white tea, fruit and herbal teas, mineral water (low sodium), red and white (dry) white wine, unsweetened fruit juices (or fresh produce for home juicing)

dairy products
plain low-fat bio yogurt, plain low-fat cottage cheese, plain low-fat fromage frais, mozzarella cheese omega-3 enriched spread semi-skimmed or skimmed cow's milk

fruit and vegetables
organic fruit: apples, bananas, berries, cherries, figs, grapes, kiwi fruit, lemons, limes, mango, melon, nectarines, oranges, papaya, peaches, pears, pineapple, red grapefruit (see caution on page 83), star fruit
organic vegetables: aubergines, broccoli, cabbage, carrots, Chinese leaves, corn on the cob, courgettes, green beans, leeks, mangetout, mushrooms, onions, peas, potatoes (waxy, new), red cabbage, shallots, spinach, sweetcorn, sweet potatoes, pak choi
organic salad ingredients: avocados, bean sprouts, celery, cucumber, iceberg lettuce, peppers, rocket, salad leaves, spring onions, tomatoes, watercress
dried fruit: apricots, dates, figs, raisins

nuts and seeds (unsalted)
almonds (whole, ground and flaked), Brazil nuts, coconut, walnuts, nut butter (such as almond), linseeds, pumpkin, sesame and sunflower seeds

herbs, spices, oils, vinegar
herbs: basil, bay leaf, chives, coriander leaf, garlic, mint, oregano, parsley, rosemary, tarragon, thyme
spices: black pepper, chillies, ground cinnamon, coriander seeds, ground cumin, curry powder, ginger root, nutmeg
oils and vinegar: extra virgin olive oil, standard olive oil, extra virgin coconut oil, walnut oil, balsamic vinegar, low-sodium soy sauce, wholegrain mustard, low-fat mayonnaise

grains
brown rice, bulgur wheat, crispbread, muesli cereals, for example, barley, bran, rye or wheat flakes (or buy unsweetened ready-made muesli), instant porridge oats, rice cakes, rolled oats, oatcakes, pitta, rye bread, wholegrain bread/rolls, wholemeal pasta

proteins
halibut, mackerel (fresh and smoked), salmon, trout (fresh and smoked), tuna (in spring water/olive oil), omega-3 rich eggs, lamb shanks, skinless chicken/turkey,

miscellaneous
organic clear honey, organic dark chocolate (at least 70 percent cocoa solids)

---

53 and 55 respectively. Also throw away foods that contain trans fats (see page 51).

The gentle program diet encourages you to eat red meat in moderation. Long-term observational studies show that a higher intake of fruit and vegetables and a lower intake of red meat can prevent increases in blood pressure with age. The occasional lean steak or lamb shank is fine, but as the World Cancer Research Fund suggests, you should limit red meat intake to no more than 80g (less than 3oz) per day.

None of the recipes in the gentle program include table salt (sodium chloride). Instead, you can add flavour to food by using fresh herbs and black pepper. At first food may taste bland, but over the course of the month you will start to notice how much better fresh, unsalted food can taste. Please do not be tempted to add salt during cooking or at the table; if you do, you will not gain the optimum benefits from this program.

Losing weight Although it's not specifically designed to be a weight-loss tool, the gentle program diet should enable you to lose any excess weight slowly and naturally. This is because you are eating healthily and avoiding high intakes of refined carbohydrates and excess fats, both of which contribute to excess weight and hypertension.

If you need to lose weight, you may wish to enhance the process by eating smaller portions and by cutting out some of the starchy foods suggested in each daily eating plan (for example, wholemeal toast, rolls, pasta, rice and couscous). Make the focus of your diet protein foods, fruit and vegetables.

The gentle program exercise routine

If you have not exercised much over the past few years, it's important to ease into regular exercise slowly to avoid aches and pains that might otherwise put you off. These daily exercise routines provide a

Gentle program supplements

I suggest you take the following supplements while you follow the gentle program. They are widely available in pharmacies, super-markets and healthfood stores. You can find information about these supplements and their blood pressure-lowering effects on pages 60–63.

recommended daily supplements

- Vitamin C (500mg)
- Vitamin E (200i.u/134mg)
- Lycopene carotenoid complex (15mg)
- Selenium (50mcg)
- Co-enzyme Q10 (60mg)
- Garlic tablets (allicin yield 1000–1500mcg)
- Omega-3 fish oil (300mg daily; for example, 1g fish oil capsule supplying 180mg EPA plus 120mg DHA)

optional daily supplements (these will provide additional health benefits)

- Alpha-lipoic acid (100mg). May be combined with L-carnitine in a 1:1 ratio
- Magnesium (300mg)
- Calcium (500mg)
- Folic acid (400mcg) plus vitamin B12 (50mcg)
- Reishi (500mg)
- Bilberry fruit extracts (60mg – standardized to give 25 percent anthocyanins)
- Probiotics (in the form of fermented milk drinks, bio yogurt or supplements)

series of stretching exercises to help limber you up and get you moving. A regular morning stretch routine will help to tone your body and relax your mind – both of which can bring your blood pressure down.

In addition, you should do some cardiovascular exercise, such as walking, for at least 15 minutes a day. You need to exercise at a rate that is brisk enough to raise your pulse rate by about 100 beats per minute (unless you are taking a beta-blocker drug; see page 24) and to make you slightly breathless.

Over the next month, you will gradually build up your cardiovascular exercise in time and intensity until you are doing 30 minutes' brisk exercise every day. As explained on page 69, you don't have to do 30 minutes' exercise all in one go – you can do three bouts of 10 minutes each if you prefer.

Walking is one of the easiest, and cheapest, ways of achieving and maintaining fitness. It is useful to buy a small pedometer to clip to your clothes. This measures the number of steps you take each day. Ideally, you need to take 10,000 steps a day. If you are unfit, aim for 5,000 steps and slowly work up to a higher target.

When starting an exercise routine, always monitor your 10-second pulse rate (see page 69) to ensure you are not overdoing it. If you have angina or a history of heart attack, ask your doctor for guidance on how much exercise you can take.

The gentle program therapies

I suggest a number of complementary therapies, such as meditation, that can reduce blood pressure. Some, such as relaxation therapies, can be practised at home, while others are practitioner-led, at least initially. Please look at days seven and fourteen of the program now so that you can make advance appointments with the appropriate therapists.

the gentle program day one

Daily menu

- **Breakfast: home-made muesli (see page 100) with almonds and blueberries**

- **Morning snack: a piece of fruit (choose from the selection on the shopping list; see page 80)**

- **Lunch: tuna, bean and pepper salad (see page 102). Small wholemeal pitta bread or granary roll**

- **Afternoon snack: low-fat bio yogurt. Handful of dried figs and almonds**

- **Dinner: baked oriental salmon (see page 103). Brown rice. Bowl of mixed salad leaves**

- **Drinks: 570ml (1pt) semi-skimmed or skimmed milk. Unsweetened fresh fruit juice. Unlimited green/ black or white tea, herbal tea and mineral water. 150ml (5fl oz) red wine or unsweetened red grape juice**

- **Supplements: see page 81**

Daily exercise routine

Over the next week, I introduce a gentle exercise routine that begins with the top of your body and works down. When you've mastered the whole routine, do it every morning when you get up. Today, do the following head/neck stretch, and go for a brisk 15–20-minute walk.

Head/neck stretch

1 Stand comfortably with feet apart and shoulders relaxed.
2 Slowly drop your head toward your left shoulder. Hold the stretch for a count of five.
3 Repeat on the right side.

Remember your supplements

Keep your supplements in the same place as your other medication. Set the alarm on a watch or mobile phone to remind you to take them. Pill containers divided into seven sections (one for every day of the week) are also useful. Fill one up every Sunday. Keep medicines away from children.

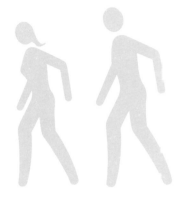

Aromatherapy

During this first week of the program, I introduce a range of relaxing ways in which to harness the therapeutic effects of aromatherapy. You will try soothing essential oils with sedative properties that can promote a better night's sleep. Sleep is important – research suggests that people with hypertension who lie awake at night have a higher blood pressure and pulse rate, and are at greater risk of heart damage than those who sleep well. Tonight, at bedtime, put 4 drops of pure lavender essential oil on a tissue and tuck it under your pillow (alternatively, use a lavender pillow or posy containing dried lavender). Lavender essential oil is gentle and suits most people.

day two

Daily menu

- **Breakfast: one red grapefruit, fresh or lightly grilled (see caution box right). Wholemeal toast with a scraping of omega-3 enriched spread or butter**

- **Morning snack: a piece of fruit**

- **Lunch: coronation turkey salad with cranberries (see page 102). Low-fat bio yogurt with fresh fruit**

- **Afternoon snack: mango and papaya smoothie (see page 109) or fresh fruit**

- **Dinner: cuban chicken (see page 104). Brown rice. Hot bananas with pumpkin seeds & lime (see page 107)**

- **Drinks: 570ml (1pt) semi-skimmed or skimmed milk. Unsweetened fresh fruit juice. Unlimited green/ black or white tea, herbal tea and mineral water. 150ml (5fl oz) red wine or unsweetened red grape juice**

- **Supplements: see page 81**

Daily exercise routine

Start with the head/neck stretch from day one and follow it with this shoulder-loosening exercise. Also walk briskly for 15–20 minutes during the day.

Shoulder loosening

1 Stand comfortably, with your feet apart. Clasp your hands behind your head.
2 Pull your elbows forward so they almost touch in front of your face. Then move your elbows out until they are as wide apart as possible.
3 Repeat several times until your shoulders have loosened up.

Aromatherapy

Have a blood pressure-lowering bath before bed. Add the following essential oils to 15ml of carrier oil (see page 29): 1 drop lavender, 2 drops geranium, 3 drops marjoram. Add the oil mixture to a warm bath, light some candles and soak for 15 minutes with your eyes closed. Before getting out, use a sponge to collect oil from the surface of the water and then massage onto your skin. Place lavender oil under your pillow as for day one.

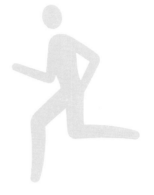

Grapefruit – eat with caution

Before you eat grapefruit, read the drug information sheet that comes with any medication you take. Grapefruit affects the absorption of some drugs, including statins and the calcium channel blocker class of anti-hypertensive drugs. This effect can be large. For example, taking one particular statin drug (lovastatin) with a glass of grapefruit juice produces the same blood levels of the drug as taking 12 tablets. If necessary, replace grapefruit with an orange – a blood orange if they are in season.

the gentle program
day three

Daily menu

- Breakfast: bircher muesli (see page 100) with a handful of mixed berries

- Morning snack: a piece of fruit

- Lunch: carrot and coriander soup (see page 101). Wholemeal roll. Bowl of mixed salad leaves. Low-fat bio yogurt with fresh fruit

- Afternoon snack: a handful of walnuts or a piece of fresh fruit

- Dinner: sliced tomato sprinkled with torn basil and olive oil. Trout with almonds and sweet potatoes (see page 106). Spinach. Sweetcorn

- Drinks: 570ml (1pt) semi-skimmed or skimmed milk. Unsweetened fresh fruit juice. Unlimited green/black or white tea, herbal tea and mineral water. 150ml (5fl oz) red wine or unsweetened red grape juice

- Supplements: see page 81

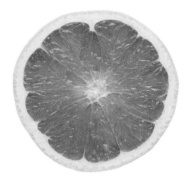

Daily exercise routine

Do the exercises from days one and two, and then add the following exercise, which mobilizes and stretches your upper body and helps to promote flexibility in your spine. For cardiovascular exercise, walk briskly for 15–20 minutes today.

Side stretch

1 Stand with your feet roughly shoulder-width apart. Slowly raise your arms above your head. Let your spine become long.
2 Bring your fingertips together above your head. Keep your shoulders relaxed.
3 Slowly lean to the right with your upper body. Feel the stretch along your left side. Now stretch to the left.

Aromatherapy

Camomile essential oil has soothing, calming properties. Put a few drops of camomile German or camomile Roman essential oil on a piece of cotton wool and place it in a small plastic box with a tightly fitting lid. Open the box and inhale the scent deeply at intervals throughout the day. Continue to use lavender essential oil under your pillow when you go to bed.

Tasty salads

To add extra flavour to today's lunchtime mixed leaf salad, sprinkle freshly chopped herbs and a little crushed garlic on the leaves. You can make a delicious dressing by combining 30ml (1fl oz) walnut oil with the juice of one lemon or lime in a screwtop jar and shaking. Walnut oil is a good source of omega-3 fatty acids, which have a thinning action on blood that helps lower blood pressure. You can further increase the omega-3 content of a salad by sprinkling it with nuts and seeds.

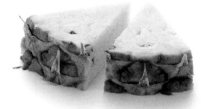

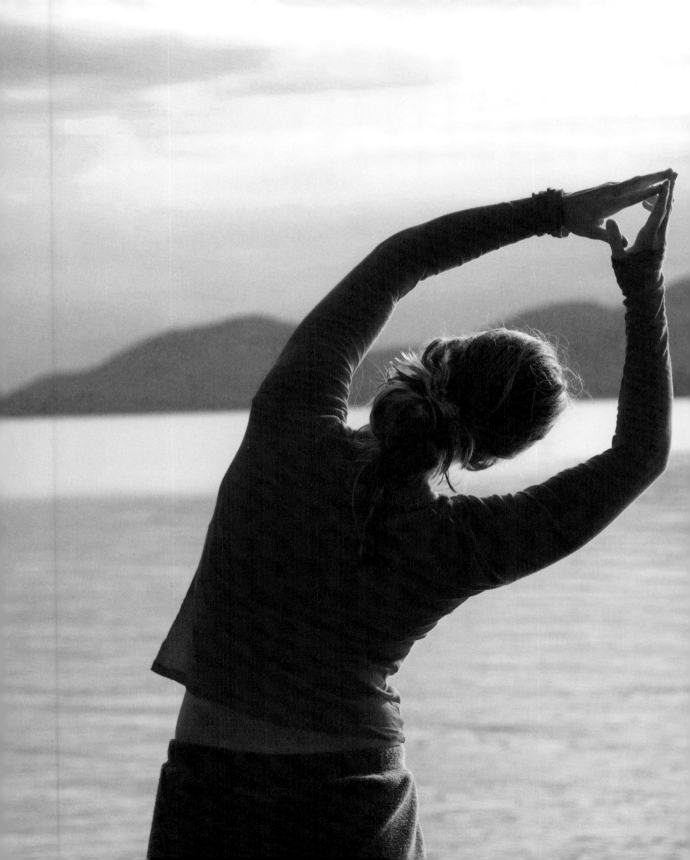

the gentle program day four

Daily menu

- **Breakfast: home-made smoothie – whizz together one small banana with 150ml (5fl oz) natural low-fat bio yogurt plus a handful of almonds**

- **Morning snack: a piece of fruit**

- **Lunch: grilled tomatoes with spinach on rye (see page 101). Bowl of mixed salad leaves drizzled with walnut oil. Low-fat bio yogurt with black grapes**

- **Afternoon snack: handful of mixed nuts**

- **Dinner: warm Mediterranean vegetable salad with balsamic dressing (see page 106). Wholemeal pasta. Bowl of mixed salad leaves. Baked peaches with raspberries (see page 108)**

- **Drinks: 570ml (1pt) semi-skimmed or skimmed milk. Unsweetened fresh fruit juice. Unlimited green/ black or white tea, herbal tea and mineral water. 150ml (5fl oz) red wine or unsweetened red grape juice**

- **Supplements: see page 81**

Having something for breakfast is very important, even if it's just a smoothie, as in today's breakfast. Researchers from Harvard Medical School have found that people who eat breakfast are 30 percent less likely to be obese than those who skip this important first meal of the day.

Daily exercise routine

Do the exercises from days one to three, and then add the following exercise. Also walk briskly for 15–20 minutes.

Forward arm stretch

1 Extend your arms in front of you at shoulder height.
2 Interlink your fingers and turn your palms outward.
3 Stretch your hands forward as far as you can and hold for 10 seconds.

Fluid intake
Lack of fluids can increase blood stickiness and may promote formation of abnormal blood clots. Don't wait until you are thirsty to drink – this is a sign of dehydration.

4 Relax, then repeat. Release your arms.

Aromatherapy
Make up a new camomile essential oil inhaling box, and inhale regularly throughout the day. In addition, start drinking camomile tea for its relaxing properties. Camomile teabags are available in supermarkets and healthfood shops. Continue to use lavender essential oil at night.

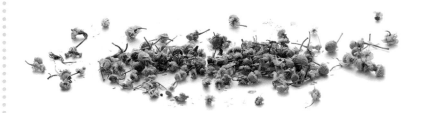

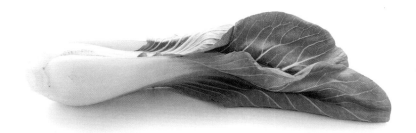

day five

daily menu

- **Breakfast: home-made muesli (see page 100)**

- **Morning snack: a piece of fruit**

- **Lunch: corn on the cob. Bowl of mixed salad leaves drizzled with walnut oil. Wholemeal roll. Low-fat bio yogurt with fresh fruit**

- **Afternoon snack: handful of grapes (preferably black or red)**

- **Dinner: bulgur wheat with peppers and bean sprouts (see page 106). Grilled chicken breast or salmon steak. Green vegetables, such as broccoli, pak choi or green beans. Low-fat fromage frais with fresh fruit**

- **Drinks: 570ml (1pt) semi-skimmed or skimmed milk. Unsweetened fresh fruit juice. Unlimited green/ black or white tea, herbal tea and mineral water. 150ml (5fl oz) red wine or unsweetened red grape juice**

- **Supplements: see page 81**

Daily exercise routine

Do the exercises from days one to four, and then add the following exercise. Also walk briskly for 15–20 minutes.

Waist twists

1 Stand comfortably with your feet apart and your hands on your hips.
2 Without moving your lower body, rotate your upper body and hips to the right, as far as you can and back again. Then rotate as far as you can to the left, then back. Repeat five times on each side.

Aromatherapy

If you spend most of the day working alone, use an essential oil burner to scent the room with a blend of anti-hypertensive essential oils. Using two or more complementary essential oils together has a synergistic effect that is more powerful than the sum of using each on their own. Use 5 drops each of marjoram, lavender and clary-sage. Alternatively, add the drops to a piece of cotton wool placed in a small plastic box that you can open and

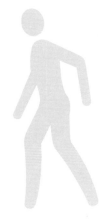

inhale regularly during the day – inhale deeply and then make your exhalation long and slow until your lungs feel empty. Breathe in and out like this two or three times. This is a good technique to use when you are feeling very stressed. Continue to use lavender essential oil to help you sleep.

Drinking less alcohol

If you drank a lot of alcohol before starting this program and are finding it difficult to cut back, you might find a supplement called kudzu (*Pueraria lobata*; see page 34) helps.

the gentle program day six

Daily menu

- **Breakfast: banana cinnamon porridge (see page 100)**

- **Morning snack: a piece of fruit**

- **Lunch: waldorf salad with red pepper (see page 102). Bowl of mixed salad leaves drizzled with walnut oil. Low-fat bio yogurt with fresh fruit**

- **Afternoon snack: handful of almonds**

- **Dinner: salmon with red pepper sauté (see page 103). Spinach. Wholemeal pasta. 40–50g (approx 1½oz) bar dark chocolate**

- **Drinks: 570ml (1pt) semi-skimmed or skimmed milk. Unsweetened fresh fruit juice. Unlimited green/ black or white tea, herbal tea and mineral water. 150ml (5fl oz) red wine or unsweetened red grape juice**

- **Supplements: see page 81**

Eating oats in the form of porridge (or muesli or oatcakes) for breakfast can help to lower your blood pressure. Recent research shows that daily consumption of whole oats can lower blood pressure by 7.5/5.5mmHg over six weeks (compared with no change in those not eating oatmeal). Researchers concluded that the soluble fibre in oatmeal is an effective dietary therapy in both the prevention and treatment of hypertension. I suggest that you include oats in your future long-term diet as much as possible.

Daily exercise routine

Do the exercises from days one to five, and then add the following exercise. Start increasing the distance you walk: spend 20–25 minutes on brisk walking today.

Forward bends

1 Stand comfortably with your feet apart.
2 Let your body curl slowly forward from your waist, keeping your legs straight, until your hands are as close to the floor as possible.
3 Touch the floor if you can.

4 Slowly straighten up. Repeat four times.

Aromatherapy

When you use the same aromatherapy oil regularly, it becomes less effective as your body adapts to its therapeutic action. So, instead of lavender oil to promote sleep, start using 2 drops each of lemongrass and orange essential oils near your pillow at night for the next five nights. From now on, change your nightly essential oil at least once a week.

Fish oil and garlic

Whenever you eat oily fish, such as salmon, I recommend adding plenty of garlic to the accompanying marinade or dressing. Fish oil and garlic have a synergistic effect. Research shows that daily garlic supplements and fish oil supplements can reduce LDL-cholesterol by 20 percent and triglycerides by 37 percent within two months. This has a blood-thinning effect that reduces hypertension.

day seven

Daily menu

- **Breakfast: grilled tomatoes on toast sprinkled with rocket and olive oil**

- **Morning snack: a piece of fruit**

- **Lunch: guacamole (see page 109). Wholemeal toast, oatcakes, rice cakes or crispbread. Bowl of mixed salad leaves drizzled with walnut oil. Low-fat bio yogurt with fresh fruit**

- **Afternoon snack: a handful of almonds**

- **Dinner: lamb shanks in red wine (see page 107). Green leafy vegetable, such as purple-sprouting broccoli or spinach. Wholemeal pasta. Poire au chocolat (see page 107)**

- **Drinks: 570ml (1pt) semi-skimmed or skimmed milk. Unsweetened fresh fruit juice. Unlimited green/ black or white tea, herbal tea and mineral water. 150ml (5fl oz) red wine or unsweetened red grape juice**

- **Supplements: see page 81**

Before you grill your tomatoes for breakfast today, drizzle them with olive oil. Cooking tomatoes in olive oil releases the most lycopene for absorption. Lycopene is an antioxidant found in tomatoes that can help lower blood pressure. The lycopene content of tomatoes is relatively small; red varieties contain the most and yellow varieties the least. The best and most concentrated source is a supplement.

Daily exercise routine

Do the exercises from days one to six, and then add the following exercise. Continue to walk briskly for 20–25 minutes today.

Thigh stretches

1 Stand comfortably, feet apart, with the back of a chair to your left. Keep your back and head straight, and your abdomen and pelvis tucked in.

2 Rest your left hand on the back of the chair for support. Bend your left knee slightly for support, then lift your right foot behind you until you can grasp your right ankle with your right hand. Keep your knees facing forward.

3 Gently ease your foot in toward your bottom until you feel a mild stretch in your thigh.

4 Hold for a count of five. Turn round and repeat the stretch on your left leg.

Consulting a homeopath

Having followed the gentle program for one week, your blood pressure should already have reduced, especially if you are taking the supplements on page 81. You may now like to consult a therapist; I suggest you start with a course of homeopathy. To find a homeopath, check the resources on page 175. A homeopath selects remedies based on your symptoms and constitutional type (of which there are 15). He or she determines your constitutional type according to your body shape, demeanour and personality. This involves answering questions about your likes, dislikes, fears, food preferences and emotions. Prescribing according to your constitutional type is important when treating a long-term condition such as hypertension, as each constitutional type has its own remedies that will work best.

the gentle program
day eight

Daily menu

- **Breakfast: low-fat bio yogurt with fresh berries**

- **Morning snack: a piece of fruit**

- **Lunch: bowl of home-made coleslaw (toss finely shredded cabbage, onion and carrot in low-fat mayonnaise). Bowl of mixed salad leaves drizzled with walnut oil. Wholemeal roll. Low-fat fromage frais with fresh fruit**

- **Afternoon snack: a handful of mixed nuts**

- **Dinner: garlic chicken (see page 103). Carrots. Spring greens. Unsweetened summer pudding (see page 108)**

- **Drinks: 570ml (1pt) semi-skimmed or skimmed milk. Unsweetened fresh fruit juice. Unlimited green/ black or white tea, herbal tea and mineral water. 150ml (5fl oz) red wine or unsweetened red grape juice**

- **Supplements: see page 81**

Daily exercise routine

Over the next week, I introduce some simple yoga poses that will help you to relax physically and mentally at the end of the day. The first is mountain pose, which helps to improve your body alignment. Continue your morning exercises (see days one to seven) and your 20–25-minute brisk walk.

Mountain pose

1 Stand with your feet slightly apart, toes facing forward.
2 Keep your back straight and your arms by your sides, palms facing inward.
3 Spread your toes and roll your pelvis forward slightly so your tailbone tucks under.
4 Pull in your tummy muscles. Tighten your pelvic floor muscles.
5 As you inhale, roll your shoulders back and down, so your chest moves forward a little.
6 Press your feet down firmly into the floor. Imagine someone is holding your hair and pulling you up from your crown.
7 Relax your upper body. Breathe in and out slowly and deeply 10 times.

Meditation

Over the next week I explain several ways of meditating that will help you switch off your body's reaction to stress. For your first meditation, sit down with your eyes shut. Imagine your favourite colour. Some people visualize colour as a dot; others as a moving cloud; others as a wash of even colour. In general, the more colour you visualize, the stronger the therapeutic effect. Focus on and explore your chosen colour. If your mind wanders, bring it back to the colour. When you feel ready, bring your mind back, open your eyes and enjoy a sense of calm.

When to avoid brisk exercise
You should avoid brisk exercise for two hours after eating a meal, and late in the evening as this may keep you awake. A gentle stroll before sleep is fine, however.

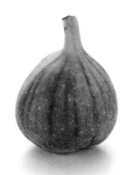

day nine

Daily menu

- **Breakfast: bircher muesli (see page 100)**

- **Morning snack: a piece of fruit**

- **Lunch: carrot and coriander soup (see page 101). Bowl of mixed salad leaves drizzled with walnut oil. Low-fat cottage cheese. Wholemeal roll. Low-fat bio yogurt with fresh fruit.**

- **Afternoon snack: a handful of Brazil nuts**

- **Dinner: Mexican spiced turkey (see page 104). Brown rice. Fresh figs**

- **Drinks: 570ml (1pt) semi-skimmed or skimmed milk. Unsweetened fresh fruit juice. Unlimited green/ black or white tea, herbal tea and mineral water. 150ml (5fl oz) red wine or unsweetened red grape juice**

- **Supplements: see page 81**

Today's dinnertime dessert is figs. Figs are an excellent source of potassium, which helps to reduce blood pressure by flushing excess sodium and fluids from the body via your kidneys. Figs are also one of the richest dietary sources of soluble fibre and help reduce cholesterol and triglyceride levels (see page 51). They are delicious eaten fresh. You can also freeze fresh figs – because they don't freeze hard, you can eat them straight from the freezer as a snack.

Daily exercise routine

Do the first yoga pose in your evening sequence (see day eight), and then do the following leg stretch. Continue to do your morning exercises (see days one to seven) and your daily 20–25-minute walk.

Wide-leg stretch

1 From the mountain pose, inhale deeply then move your feet wide apart and point your toes comfortably inward. Put your hands on your hips and, as you slowly breathe out, bend forward from your hips, keeping your spine straight.

2 Keep your legs straight, push down through your feet and lift your tailbone. Keep your chest facing forward.

3 Try to lengthen your spine as much as possible. Hold the stretch for five slow, deep breaths.

Meditation

Today, weather permitting, I'd like you to sit in a shady, private spot outdoors, perhaps in your garden or a park. Close your eyes and immerse yourself in the relaxing qualities of nature for 10–20 minutes. Try to isolate all the different sounds you can hear – insects buzzing, birds singing, wind rustling in the trees. Notice the way the light intensity on your eyelids varies with the dappling effects of leaves and moving clouds. Focus on the breeze caressing your skin, or the sun's warmth. Smell the damp, earthy or warm herby odours around you. If thoughts of life and work intrude, gently bring your awareness back to your contemplation of your surroundings. When you are ready, stand up, breathe in deeply and stretch. Now enjoy your day.

10

the gentle program day ten

Daily menu

- **Breakfast: home-made muesli (see page 100). Low-fat bio yogurt**

- **Morning snack: a piece of fruit**

- **Lunch: smoked trout and lemon pâté (see page 109). Wholemeal toast or oatcakes. Rocket. Low-fat bio yogurt with mango cubes**

- **Afternoon snack: a handful of mixed nuts**

- **Dinner: Cuban chicken (see page 104). Roast baby vine tomatoes. Bowl of mixed salad leaves drizzled with walnut oil. Hot bananas with pumpkin seeds and lime (see page 107)**

- **Drinks: 570ml (1pt) semi-skimmed or skimmed milk. Unsweetened fresh fruit juice. Unlimited green/ black or white tea, herbal tea and mineral water. 150ml (5fl oz) red wine or unsweetened red grape juice**

- **Supplements: see page 81**

Daily exercise routine

Do the first two yoga poses in your evening sequence (see days eight and nine), and then add the following pose. Continue to do your morning exercises (see days one to seven), and your daily 20–25-minute walk.

Downward dog

1 Start on all fours with your knees together and your hands firmly on the floor, shoulder-width apart.

2 Lift your knees off the ground and push your tailbone high in the air so your body makes a wide inverted "V" shape. Your arms and legs should be straight.

3 Pull your tummy in toward your spine and lift your pelvic floor muscles. Press your heels and the palms of your hands into the floor. Don't let them slide away. Let your spine become long. Hold this posture for five slow, deep breaths, then relax.

Meditation

Yesterday, you sat in quiet contemplation with nature. Today, I'd like you to sit quietly and focus on your body. Breathe in and out slowly and deeply. Be mindful of what happens when you breathe. Follow the passage of air through your nostrils or lips. Observe how your abdomen rises as you inhale, and falls as you exhale, and how your ribcage expands to pull air into your body, then contracts to push air out. Note whether your breath is shallow or deep, smooth or ragged. Focus on your circulation. Become aware of your heart beating and blood pulsing through your arteries.

The more you focus on your body, the more you switch off from the world. Do this for 15 minutes or as long as you like.

A vegetarian diet

People who follow a vegetarian diet tend to have a systolic blood pressure that is around 5mmHg lower than meat eaters. This reduction occurs within six weeks of omitting meat from the diet (and blood pressure rises to its previous levels within six weeks of eating meat again).

92 the natural health guru programs

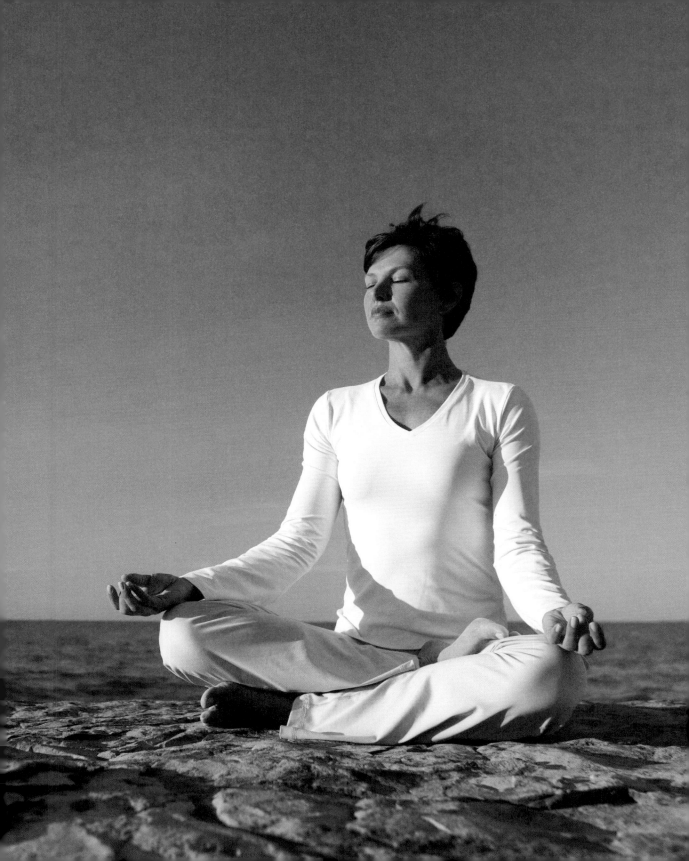

the gentle program day eleven

Daily menu

- **Breakfast: frittata (see page 101). Rocket. Wholemeal toast**

- **Morning snack: orange and carrot juice (see page 109)**

- **Lunch: tuna, bean and pepper salad (see page 102). Wholemeal roll or oatcake. Low-fat bio yogurt with fresh fruit**

- **Afternoon snack: a handful of mixed nuts**

- **Dinner: halibut with tarragon sauce (see page 104). Sweetcorn. Spinach. A handful of red or black grapes**

- **Drinks: 570ml (1pt) semi-skimmed or skimmed milk. Unsweetened fresh fruit juice. Unlimited green/ black or white tea, herbal tea and mineral water. 150ml (5fl oz) red wine or unsweetened red grape juice**

- **Supplements: see page 81**

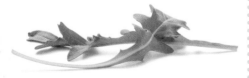

Make today's breakfast with omega-3 enriched eggs. Research shows that eating four enriched eggs a week for four weeks not only significantly reduces your systolic blood pressure, it also lowers your triglyceride level (and does not raise your cholesterol levels).

Daily exercise routine

Do the first three yoga poses in your evening sequence (see days eight to ten), and then add the following pose. Continue to do your morning exercises (see days one to seven) and your daily 20–25-minute brisk walk.

The plank

1 From downward dog (see day ten) lower your bottom so your legs, back and head form a straight line – like a plank.

2 Gently tuck your chin in and look at the floor. Let your weight rest on your toes and palms (spread your fingers and thumbs). Pull your tummy in toward your spine and squeeze your pelvic floor muscles.

3 Maintain this pose for five slow, deep breaths.

Eat more carrots

Carrots contain substances called cumarin glycosides that reduce arterial blood pressure through actions similar to that of calcium channel blockers (see page 24).

Meditation

By focusing your mind on a particular object, such as a mandala, you can screen out distractions and, with time and practice, you can enter a state of profound relaxation and serenity. A mandala is a diagram whose name derives from the Sanskrit word for "circle".

Today, I'd like you to find a mandala and spend 15 minutes focusing on it. You can search for mandalas on the internet or create your own using colours and shapes that please you – look in books or online for inspiration. (You can also gaze at the patterns in a child's kaleidoscope.) During your contemplation, let your gaze wander over the shapes and angles of the mandala. Absorb the colours and patterns into your mind.

day twelve

Daily menu

- **Breakfast: home-made muesli (see page 100) with kiwi fruit**

- **Morning snack: a piece of fruit**

- **Lunch: carrot and coriander soup (see page 101). Wholemeal roll. Bowl of mixed salad leaves drizzled with walnut oil. Low-fat bio yogurt with fresh fruit**

- **Afternoon snack: a handful of mixed nuts**

- **Dinner: smoked mackerel mixed with mango cubes and piled onto mixed salad leaves. 40–50g (approx 1½oz) bar dark chocolate**

- **Drinks: 570ml (1pt) semi-skimmed or skimmed milk. Unsweetened fresh fruit juice. Unlimited green/ black or white tea, herbal tea and mineral water. 150ml (5fl oz) red wine or unsweetened red grape juice**

- **Supplements: see page 81**

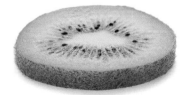

The mackerel in today's lunch is a rich source of omega-3 fatty acids; it provides twice as much as herrings. There also appears to be something special about mackerel in that it reduces renin activity (see page 13) by more than 60 per cent. So, when buying oily fish, make mackerel your first choice.

Daily exercise routine

Do the first four yoga poses in your evening sequence (see days eight to eleven), and then add the following pose. Continue to do your morning exercises (see days one to seven) and, from today, increase your daily walk to 25–30 minutes.

Four-limb staff pose

1 From plank pose, slowly bend your arms and lower your body until it's close to the floor. Squeeze your elbows in to your ribcage. Pull your tummy toward your spine, lift your pelvic floor muscles and tuck in your chin. Lengthen your spine.

2 Hover a little way off the floor with only your toes and hands in contact with the ground. Hold this stick-like posture for five slow, deep breaths.

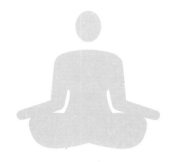

Meditation

Select an aromatherapy candle with a relaxing scent such as lavender, geranium or lemongrass (for more about the qualities of different essential oils, see page 30). Sit in a quiet room, on the floor or at a table. Light the candle and place it on a plate a short distance away from you.

Focus on the flame. Look deeply into it. Explore it and watch how it flickers in front of you. As thoughts enter your head, notice them and then just quietly let them go again. Keep returning your attention to the flame. After a while, close your eyes and watch the flame dance in your mind's eye. If the image starts to fade, just open your eyes to look at the flame again. Do this meditation for up to 20 minutes before safely extinguishing the flame.

the gentle program day thirteen

Daily menu

- **Breakfast: fresh fruit smoothie (see day four). Wholemeal toast**

- **Morning snack: a piece of fruit**

- **Lunch: pear, avocado and nut salad (see page 102). Bowl of mixed salad leaves drizzled with walnut oil. Low-fat bio yogurt with fresh fruit**

- **Afternoon snack: smoked trout and lemon pâté (see page 109)**

- **Dinner: slice of melon. Bulgur wheat with peppers and bean sprouts (see page 106). Grilled chicken or salmon steak**

- **Drinks: 570ml (1pt) semi-skimmed or skimmed milk. Unsweetened fresh fruit juice. Unlimited green/ black or white tea, herbal tea and mineral water. 150ml (5fl oz) red wine or unsweetened red grape juice**

- **Supplements: see page 81**

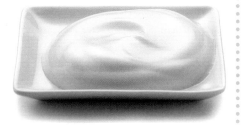

You should be in the habit of eating bio yogurt every day by now. Bio yogurt contains probiotic bacteria that break down milk proteins. During this process, substances known as peptides are produced, which have anti-hypertensive properties.

Daily exercise routine

Do the first five yoga poses in your evening sequence (see days eight to twelve), and then add the cobra. Continue to do your morning exercises (see days one to seven) and walk for 25–30 minutes.

The cobra

1 From the four-limb staff pose, let your body drop gently to the floor.
2 Let your legs relax and your toes point out behind you.
3 With your hands just under your shoulders, lift your head, neck and upper chest, keeping your head in line with your spine. Keep your hips on the floor and your legs relaxed.
4 Look forward and up while supporting your weight on your palms. Maintain this posture for five slow, deep breaths.

Crystal meditation

Crystals can greatly enhance the power of a meditation. Select a crystal you feel particularly drawn to, or choose from those traditionally used to reduce blood pressure and induce relaxation: amethyst (calming and relaxing); aventurine (increases creativity and reduces hypertension); sodalite (boosts endurance and helps to reduce hypertension); or prehnite (used where hypertension is associated with kidney problems).

Sit comfortably in a quiet room and hold your chosen crystal in your hands. Close your eyes and try to picture the crystal in your mind's eye. Let the colours, shapes and textures of the crystal swirl through your mind, as it draws you deeper down into a quiet, relaxing space.

If your mind wanders, open your eyes and gaze at the crystal, exploring its shape. It is surprisingly easy to imagine yourself inside the crystal exploring its many facets. In your own time, bring the meditation to a close – around 20 minutes is a good length of time to spend on this relaxing therapy.

day fourteen

Daily menu

- **Breakfast: banana cinnamon porridge (see page 100)**

- **Morning snack: a piece of fruit**

- **Lunch: coronation turkey salad with cranberries (see page 102). Bowl of mixed salad leaves drizzled with walnut oil. Wholemeal roll. Low-fat bio yogurt with fresh fruit**

- **Afternoon snack: fruit smoothie**

- **Dinner: half an avocado sprinkled with chopped walnuts. Baked Oriental salmon (see page 103). Broccoli. Carrots**

- **Drinks: 570ml (1pt) semi-skimmed or skimmed milk. Unsweetened fresh fruit juice. Unlimited green/ black or white tea, herbal tea and mineral water. 150ml (5fl oz) red wine or unsweetened red grape juice**

- **Supplements: see page 81**

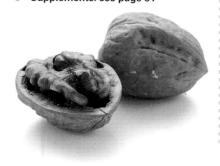

Daily exercise routine

Do the first six yoga poses in your evening sequence (see days eight to thirteen), and then add the corpse pose. Continue to do your morning exercises (see days one to seven) and walk for 25–30 minutes. From now on, try to walk briskly for at least 30 minutes on most days of the week. To add variety to your cardiovascular exercise routine, try replacing walking with swimming, dancing or cycling on some days.

The corpse pose

1   Lie on your back with your arms out to the sides and your palms facing upward. Start with your feet pointing up, then let your hips rotate so your feet drop comfortably out to either side.

2   Close your eyes and allow every muscle in your body to relax as if you are sinking into the floor. Mentally scan your body for any remaining pockets of tension.

3   Breathe slowly and softly, and try to feel the flow of energy through your body. Stay in this posture for 5–10 minutes.

Consulting an aromatherapist

Now you are at the end of the program, I suggest you try a relaxing and therapeutic aromatherapy massage. To find an aromatherapist, check the resources at the end of this book (see page 174). An aromatherapist will select essential oils that help to lower blood pressure and encourage you to relax. During your first session, he or she will ask questions about your medical history and lifestyle. The therapist may select the oils themselves or invite you to choose your preferred aromas from a selection. Aromatherapy massage is usually based on Swedish massage techniques and may also involve acupressure. A full-body massage lasts around 60 minutes. You will feel relaxed and, often, sleepy afterwards. An aromatherapist may supply oils for you to take home and inhale or massage into your skin. A medical aromatherapist may also prescribe aromatherapy oils for internal use – never consume aromatherapy oils except under professional supervision. If you enjoy the massage, book yourself in for four weekly sessions.

continuing the gentle program

You have now followed the gentle program for two weeks – congratulations! I suggest that you continue with the eating plan for a further two weeks. This way you will have a month of healthy eating behind you, and you will be very familiar with the foods you need to shop for and eat every day. You can vary the foods you eat, and include some new recipes. You will find some new recipe suggestions at www.naturalhealth-guru.co.uk. You can also post your own favourites there for other followers of the plan to try. The information below will help you map out your future using the principles of the gentle program.

Your long-term diet

The gentle program provides a simple diet based on healthy, low-glycemic principles such as those described in the DASH diet (see page 46). This encourages you to eat plenty of wholegrains, fruits, vegetables, low-fat dairy products, fish, poultry, nuts and beans, while cutting back on red meat, sweets, saturated fats and sodium. Continue to eat according to these principles. This checklist enables you to see at a glance what you should be eating each day:

- At least five (and preferably eight to 10) servings of fruit, vegetables and saladstuff.
- Two to eight servings of wholegrains. One serving is equivalent to one slice of wholemeal bread or 100g (3½oz/½ cup) of cooked brown rice or wholemeal pasta.
- Two to three servings of low-fat dairy products.

- No more than two servings of meat/fish/poultry/ eggs (ideally no more than 85g/3oz lean meat per serving). Select omega-3 enriched hen's eggs wherever possible as, unlike normal hen's eggs, these have beneficial effects on your blood pressure and blood cholesterol levels.
- At least one serving of nuts, seeds or beans.

Adapting recipes You can usually adapt recipes from any cookery writer to meet the principles of the gentle program. Here are some guidelines:

- Omit salt or sugar from recipes. You can add honey occasionally if additional sweetness is desirable.
- Make food tasty by adding lots of freshly chopped herbs. If you have space in your garden or on your windowsill to grow herbs, this can become a rewarding hobby.
- Replace single cream with low-fat natural yogurt, and double cream with fromage frais. Experiment to see what works best.
- Add yogurt to sauces or casseroles off the heat, and don't add yogurt to liquids at boiling point – the mixture may curdle. This won't affect the flavour, but it looks unsightly. Creamy Greek yogurt has a higher fat content than regular yogurt and is more stable – so it may suit some recipes better than thinner yogurts.
- You can make yogurt less likely to curdle by stabilizing it. Stir in one teaspoon of cornflour per 150m (5fl oz) yogurt before using it in a recipe.

- Rather than using yogurt as a topping for baked dishes, use fromage frais (yogurt protein coagulates). Alternatively, add yogurt (mixed with herbs and seasoning) after the dish is out of the oven.

Your long-term supplement regime

Continue taking the recommended supplements for the gentle program (see page 81) long term. Research supports their use at this level for gentle yet significant effects on blood pressure and future health. If, until now, you have taken only the supplements in the recommended list, you may wish to add in one or more of the supplements in the optional list for additional benefits. Go to pages 60–63 to read more about the supplements in which you are interested.

Your exercise routine

After just two weeks of regular exercise you should have started to notice a difference in your fitness level. Continue with your morning exercise regime at the beginning of the day. Fit in at least 30 minutes of brisk exercise during the day. This can be walking, cycling, swimming, dancing or gardening – whatever activity you enjoy. Vary the type of exercise you do from day to day. Then, at the end of each day, do the wind-down yoga sequence to lower your blood pressure and relax you in preparation for a good night's sleep.

Your therapy program

The gentle program has shown you how to use aromatherapy and meditation for relaxation. Although these activities may seem simple, don't underestimate the powerful effect they can have on your cardiovascular health and general well-being. Try to practise one relaxation technique each day – or combine the two therapies by meditating while scenting the room with essential oils. If you found homeopathy and aromatherapy useful, continue sessions on a regular basis.

Burn off calories by walking

Exercise can burn a surprising number of calories and will help to keep your weight down, as well as your blood pressure. For example, walking briskly (7.2 kilometres per hour/4½ miles per hour) for 30 minutes burns 200 calories. Walking is an ideal form of exercise if you have previously been inactive for a long time. You can start very gently and build up the intensity as your fitness levels improve.

Monitoring your blood pressure

I suggest you monitor your blood pressure on a weekly basis, at the same time of day each time, unless your doctor has asked you to check it more frequently. Record your blood pressure measurements in a chart such as the one on page 77. This will give you an instant visual indication of whether your blood pressure is going down (as it should during this program), staying the same, or going up.

If your blood pressure is consistently below 130/80mmHg, well done – this program has worked well for you. You may now want to discuss with your doctor the ways in which your treatment can change to reflect your lower blood pressure. It's important to be aware, however, that the dose of some anti-hypertensive drugs must be reduced slowly to prevent any rebound effects in which your blood pressure quickly bounces back up again.

If your blood pressure is consistently between 130/80mmHg and 140/90mmHg, consider moving up to the moderate program (see pages 111–141) to see if you can bring it down to below 130/80mmHg. If your blood pressure is consistently above 140/90mmHg, move onto the moderate program, but consult your doctor for individual advice.

breakfast recipes

home-made muesli

serves 4

1 handful rolled oats
3 handfuls mixed cereals (toasted
    wheat, rye, barley and bran flakes)
1 handful mixed nuts, such as walnuts,
    Brazil nuts and flaked almonds,
    roughly chopped
1 handful mixed seeds, such as sun-
    flower, pumpkin and sesame seeds
1 handful raisins or sultanas
1 handful chopped apricots, dates or
    figs (optional)
Milk, to serve

1 Mix together all the ingredients
    except the milk in a large bowl.
2 Divide between four serving
    bowls and pour over enough
    milk to taste.

banana cinnamon porridge

serves 4

600ml/1pt/2½ cups water
150g/5½oz/1½ cups instant
    porridge oats
1 tsp freshly ground cinnamon
1 large banana, sliced

1 Bring the water to boiling point
    in a medium saucepan. Add the
    porridge oats and a good sprin-
    kling of the cinnamon. Simmer
    gently, stirring continuously, for
    about 1 minute. Remove from
    the heat, cover and leave for
    at least 5 minutes, until all the
    liquid has been absorbed.
2 Divide between four serving
    bowls and top with the banana
    and the remaining
    cinnamon.

bircher muesli

serves 4

1 sweet apple
Grated zest and freshly squeezed juice
    of 1 unwaxed lemon
350g/12oz/2 cups rolled oats
600ml/1pt/2½ cups semi-skimmed,
    soy or almond milk (or low-fat bio
    yogurt)
100g/3½oz/⅔ cup raisins
1 banana, thinly sliced
1 orange, peeled and roughly chopped
1 handful chopped nuts
1 handful fresh seasonal fruit, such as
    berries, peaches, nectarines, pears
    or cherries, roughly chopped if
    necessary, to serve

1 Peel and core the apple. Grate
    into a bowl, then sprinkle over
    the lemon juice and zest (to
    prevent the apple discolouring).
2 Add the oats, milk, raisins,
    banana and orange flesh and
    mix well. Cover and leave in
    the fridge overnight.
3 Divide between four serving
    bowls. Serve with a topping
    of chopped nuts and fresh
    seasonal fruit.

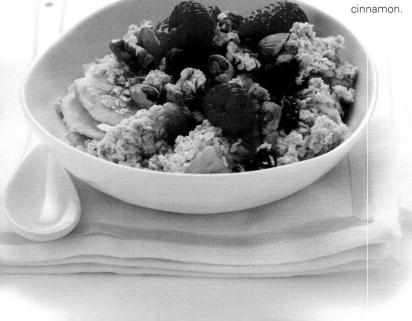

bircher muesli

lunch recipes

frittata

serves 4

8 organic omega-3 enriched eggs
½ tbsp olive oil
2 shallots, sliced
2 cloves garlic, crushed
1 red or orange pepper, sliced
3 large handfuls fresh spinach, washed
   and roughly chopped
4 medium tomatoes, sliced
1 handful fresh basil leaves, torn
Freshly ground black pepper
1 small bunch watercress, to serve

1 Preheat the grill to hot. Beat
   the eggs well and season to
   taste with black pepper. Set on
   one side.
2 Heat a non-stick frying pan until
   hot. Add the oil, then the shallots, garlic and red pepper and
   sauté over a medium heat for
   5 minutes. Pour over the egg
   mixture, then scatter over the
   spinach, tomatoes and basil.
   Cook on a low heat,
   without stirring, for 3 minutes.
3 Put the pan under the hot grill
   and leave until the top of the
   frittata is golden brown. Serve,
   garnished with sprigs of
   watercress.

carrot and coriander soup

serves 4

½ tbsp olive oil
1 onion, finely chopped
2 garlic cloves, crushed
450g/1lb carrots, grated
   or finely chopped, plus one carrot,
   grated, to serve
1 tbsp coriander seeds, crushed or
   ground
750ml/1½pt/3 cups vegetable stock (see
   page 109) or water
Freshly squeezed lemon juice, to taste
100ml/3½fl oz/^{1}/$_3$ cup low-fat
   bio yogurt
1 handful fresh coriander leaves,
   roughly chopped
Pinch of nutmeg, grated (optional)
Freshly ground black pepper

1 Heat the oil in a large pan. Add
   the onion and garlic and cook
   gently until soft.
2 Add the carrots, coriander
   seeds and stock and bring to
   the boil. Reduce the heat and
   simmer for 20 minutes. Allow
   to cool a little, then purée in
   a blender. Season with black
   pepper and lemon juice.
3 Return to the pan and heat
   gently. Serve topped with
   yogurt, grated carrot, chopped
   coriander and nutmeg, if using.

grilled tomatoes with spinach on rye

serves 4

4 large slices rye bread
Extra virgin olive oil or walnut oil,
   for drizzling
3 large handfuls spinach leaves,
   washed and wilted in a steamer
4 ripe medium tomatoes, thinly sliced
4 thin slices mozzarella cheese
   (optional)
Freshly ground black pepper

1 Preheat the grill to hot, then
   lightly toast the rye bread on
   both sides.
2 Remove from the grill and
   drizzle a little oil over each
   piece of toast. Arrange the
   spinach and tomatoes on top.
   Drizzle over a little more
   oil or, if preferred, top with
   mozzarella cheese. Season to
   taste with black pepper.
3 Return to the hot grill for a few
   minutes, until lightly brown or
   the cheese is melted. Serve
   immediately.

tuna, bean and pepper salad

serves 4

400g/14oz tin mixed beans, drained
200g/7oz tin tuna in spring water or
    olive oil (not brine), drained
1 red pepper, deseeded and chopped
1 green pepper, deseeded and chopped
1 red onion, finely chopped
1 handful fresh flat-leaf parsley, finely
    chopped

For the dressing:
2 tbsp extra virgin olive oil or walnut oil
2 tbsp red wine vinegar
1 garlic clove, crushed
Freshly ground black pepper

1   Mix the beans, tuna, chopped
    peppers, red onion and parsley
    together in a large serving bowl.
2   To make the dressing, put
    the oil, vinegar and garlic in
    a screw-top jar. Shake, and
    season with black pepper. Pour
    the dressing over the
    salad and toss well.

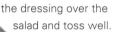

coronation turkey salad with cranberries

serves 4

1 large handful dried cranberries
4 tbsp red wine vinegar
½ tbsp olive oil
3 tsp curry powder
1 iceberg lettuce, shredded
150ml/5fl oz/½ cup low-fat bio yogurt or
    fromage frais
450g/1lb cooked turkey breast, cubed
1 medium carrot, grated
1 cucumber, deseeded and finely
    chopped
1 handful fresh coriander leaves, finely
    chopped
3 tbsp flaked almonds
Freshly ground black pepper

1   Microwave the dried cranber-
    ries and vinegar on a high
    setting for 90 seconds.
2   Heat the oil in a pan, add the
    curry powder and stir-fry for 1
    minute. Add the cranberries
    and vinegar and stir-fry for a
    further minute. Transfer to a
    large bowl and put in the fridge
    for about 5 minutes. Put the
    lettuce in a large serving bowl.
3   Mix the yogurt with the cooled
    cranberry mixture. Season
    with black pepper. Fold in the
    turkey, carrot, cucumber and
    coriander leaves. Pile on top of
    the lettuce. Sprinkle over the
    flaked almonds and serve.

waldorf salad with red pepper

serves 4

4 red apples, peeled, cored and
    chopped
Grated zest and freshly squeezed juice
    of 1 unwaxed lemon
150ml/5fl oz/½ cup low-fat fromage frais
4 celery stalks, chopped
1 red pepper, deseeded and chopped
100g/3½oz/1 cup walnut halves
1 iceberg lettuce, shredded
1 handful fresh parsley, chopped
Freshly ground black pepper

1   Mix all the ingredients except
    the lettuce and parsley.
2   Pile the mixture on top of the
    lettuce. Sprinkle with parsley.

pear, avocado and nut salad

serves 4

150ml/5fl oz/½ cup low-fat fromage frais
Grated zest and freshly squeezed juice
    of 1 unwaxed lemon
3 tsp white wine vinegar
1 handful fresh chives, chopped
2 avocados, peeled, stoned and sliced
1 pear, peeled, cored and chopped
Salad leaves
8 walnut halves
1 handful flaked almonds
Freshly ground black pepper

1   Mix all the ingredients except
    the leaves and nuts. Season.
2   Pile the mixture on top of the
    leaves. Sprinkle with nuts.

dinner recipes

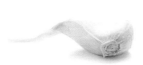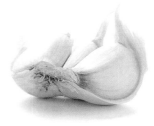

garlic chicken

serves 4

1 onion, chopped
4 celery sticks, chopped
2 carrots, chopped
1 small red pepper, deseeded and
  chopped
1 sprig thyme
1 sprig rosemary
1 handful fresh basil leaves, torn
1 bay leaf
2 garlic bulbs, with individual cloves
  peeled but not separated from the
  bulb
4 skinless chicken breasts, about
  200g/7oz each
100ml/3½fl oz/1 glass medium-dry
  white wine
Freshly ground black pepper
Crusty wholemeal bread, to serve
  (optional)

1 Preheat the oven to
  180°C/350°F/Gas 4.
2 Put the vegetables, herbs and
  garlic in an oven-proof dish.
  Add the chicken and wine and
  season with black pepper.
  Cover and bake for 1½ hours.
3 Remove the garlic from the
  casserole. Cover the casserole
  and keep it warm. Squeeze the
  garlic paste from the cloves
  onto slices of bread. Serve with
  the casserole, if you like.

baked oriental salmon

serves 4

4 salmon fillets
4 spring onions, shredded
1 small red pepper, deseeded and thinly
  sliced
5cm/2in piece fresh ginger, peeled and
  grated
1 handful fresh coriander leaves,
  roughly chopped
4 tbsp olive oil
Freshly squeezed juice of 1 lime
1 tbsp low-sodium soy sauce
1 tsp clear honey (optional)
Freshly ground black pepper

1 Preheat the oven to
  180°C/350°F/Gas 4.
2 Put a large sheet of foil in a
  shallow baking dish. Lay the
  salmon fillets in a single layer
  in the middle. Sprinkle over
  the spring onions, red pepper,
  ginger and coriander leaves.
3 Mix the oil, lime juice, soy
  sauce and honey (if using).
  Season, then pour the mixture
  over the fish. Wrap the foil over
  the fish and seal well.
4 Bake in the oven for 45 minutes. Unwrap the salmon and
  place on warm serving plates.
  Pour over any juices left in the
  foil and serve.

salmon with red pepper sauté

serves 4

4 salmon fillets
½ tbsp olive oil
1 small handful fresh basil, dill or
  parsley, roughly chopped

For the red pepper sauté:
1 tsp olive oil
1 onion, thinly sliced
2 garlic cloves, crushed
2 red peppers, deseeded and chopped
100ml/3½fl oz/1 glass dry white wine
Freshly ground black pepper

1 Preheat the oven to
  180°C/350°F/Gas 4.
2 Put the salmon in a shallow
  baking dish. Brush with oil and
  season with pepper. Bake for
  20 minutes or until cooked.
3 Meanwhile, prepare the sauté.
  Heat a wok until hot. Add the
  oil and swirl it around. Stir-fry
  the onion and garlic for 5 minutes. Add the red pepper and
  stir-fry for another 5 minutes.
  Pour in the wine and cook for a
  further 5 minutes or until most
  of the liquid evaporates.
4 Divide the sauté between four
  plates. Top each with a salmon
  fillet. Sprinkle with herbs.

mexican spiced turkey

serves 4

4 tbsp blanched almonds
6 tbsp sesame seeds
6 tbsp raisins
1–2 red chillies, deseeded
2 garlic cloves, crushed
2 tsp ground cinnamon
1 tsp ground cumin
1 onion, chopped
4 large tomatoes, skinned, deseeded
　　and chopped
2 tbsp olive oil
350ml/12fl oz/1½ cups vegetable stock
　　(see page 109) or water
30g/1oz dark chocolate, grated
1kg/2lb 4oz skinless turkey breast, cut
　　into bite-sized cubes
1 handful fresh coriander leaves,
　　roughly chopped
Freshly ground black pepper

1　Preheat the oven to
　　180°C/350°F/Gas 4.
2　Toast the almonds and sesame
　　seeds by tossing them in a dry
　　frying pan over medium heat.
　　Grind in a blender with the
　　raisins, chillies, garlic, cinnamon
　　and cumin. Add the onion and
　　tomatoes and whizz in blender.
3　Heat the oil in a pan, add the
　　sauce and cook for 5 minutes.
　　Stir in the stock and chocolate.
　　Season with pepper.
4　Put the turkey in an oven-proof
　　dish and pour over the sauce.
　　Cover and bake for 45 minutes.
　　Stir in the coriander. Serve.

cuban chicken

serves 4

4 skinless chicken breasts
Freshly squeezed juice of 2 large
　　unwaxed preferably Seville oranges,
　　plus strips of zest, to serve
Freshly squeezed juice of 1 lime
1 tsp olive oil
2 garlic cloves, crushed
1 handful fresh herbs, such as parsley,
　　coriander and mint, roughly chopped
1 small red chilli, deseeded
　　and finely chopped
1 handful rocket
¼ large cucumber, sliced
Freshly ground black pepper

1　Preheat the oven to
　　180°C/350°F/Gas 4.
2　Put the chicken in a single layer
　　in a shallow oven-proof dish.
　　Mix the remaining ingredients,
　　except the rocket and cucum-
　　ber, and pour over the chicken.
　　Marinate for 1 hour.
3　Bake for 25 minutes or until
　　cooked. Serve with orange zest
　　and rocket and cucumber salad.

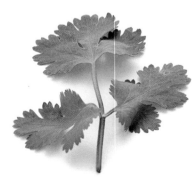

halibut with tarragon sauce

serves 4

1l/35fl oz/4 cups vegetable stock
　　(see page 109) or water
400g/14oz new potatoes, scrubbed and
　　thickly sliced
450g/1lb mixed green vegetables, such
　　as broccoli, green beans, mangetout,
　　sliced courgettes and peas
150ml/5fl oz/½ cup low-fat fromage frais
1 handful fresh tarragon, roughly
　　chopped
Freshly ground black pepper
4 halibut fillets, about 200g/7oz each

1　Preheat the oven to
　　180°C/350°F/Gas 4.
2　Pour the stock into a large
　　saucepan and bring to the boil.
　　Add the potato and cook gently
　　for 10 minutes. Remove the
　　potato and arrange in the base
　　of an oven-proof dish. Reserve
　　the stock. Scatter the green
　　vegetables over the potato.
3　Mix the fromage frais and
　　tarragon with some of the
　　reserved stock to make a thick
　　sauce. Season with pepper and
　　pour over the vegetables. Lay
　　the fish in a single layer on top,
　　then cover and bake for 30
　　minutes. Serve.

right: cuban chicken

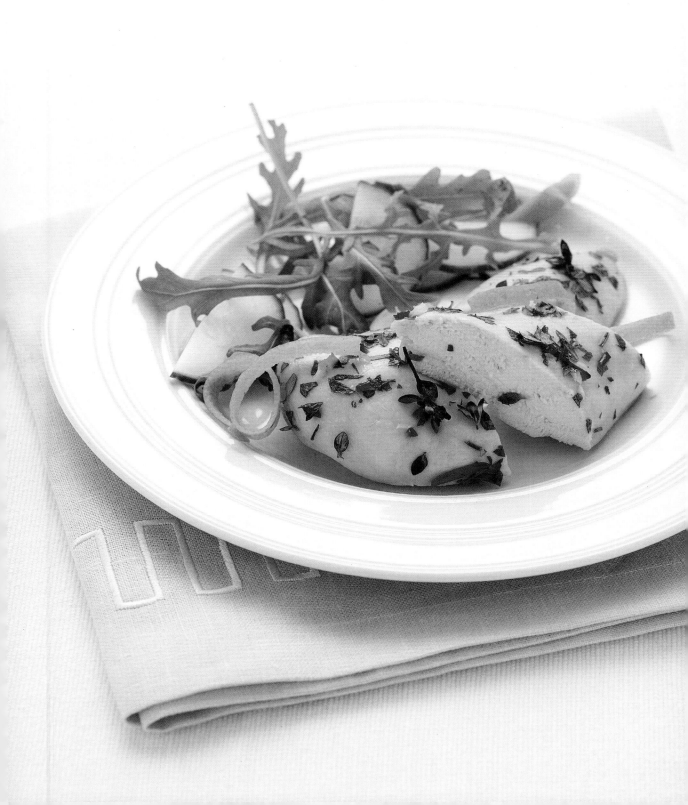

bulgur wheat with peppers and bean sprouts

serves 4

200g/7oz bulgur wheat
1.2l/2pt vegetable stock (page 109)
1 red pepper, deseeded and thinly sliced
1 green pepper, deseeded and thinly sliced
1 yellow pepper, deseeded and thinly sliced
4 medium tomatoes, thinly sliced
1 handful bean sprouts
1 red chilli, deseeded and chopped
1 handful mixed fresh herbs, such as flat-leaf parsley and mint
Grated zest and freshly squeezed juice of 1 unwaxed lemon
Freshly ground black pepper

1 Mix the ingredients in a large pan and simmer gently until the liquid has been absorbed.
2 Serve hot or cold.

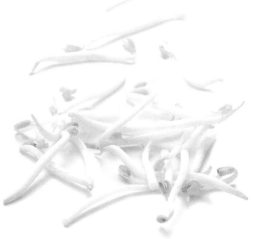

trout with almonds and sweet potatoes

serves 4

4 small sweet potatoes, scrubbed and cut into thick wedges
1 handful flaked almonds
2 tbsp olive oil
2 tbsp red wine vinegar
4 rainbow trout fillets, brushed with olive oil
Grated zest and freshly squeezed juice of 1 large orange
Grated zest and freshly squeezed juice of ½ unwaxed lemon
1 handful flat-leaf parsley, roughly chopped
Freshly ground black pepper

1 Preheat the oven to 180°C/350°F/Gas 4.
2 Put the sweet potato, almonds, oil and vinegar in a bowl and mix. Season with black pepper. Transfer to a large roasting tin and bake for 20 minutes.
3 Take the tin out of the oven and push the sweet potato and almonds to one end. Put each trout fillet in the middle of a piece of foil. Sprinkle the orange and lemon juices and zest over the fish, then seal in the foil. Put the parcels in the free end of the roasting tin. Return the tin to the oven for 20 minutes or until cooked.
4 Sprinkle with the chopped parsley and serve.

warm mediterranean vegetable salad with balsamic dressing

serves 4

For the balsamic dressing:
5 tbsp balsamic vinegar
5 tbsp extra virgin olive oil
1 tsp wholegrain mustard
3 garlic cloves, crushed
1 sprig rosemary, leaves roughly chopped
Freshly ground black pepper

1 red onion, cut into 8 wedges
2 courgettes, quartered lengthways
8 cherry tomatoes, cut in half
1 red pepper, deseeded and chopped
1 yellow pepper, deseeded and chopped
1 green pepper, deseeded and chopped
250g/9oz rocket or mixed baby salad leaves
1 handful fresh parsley, roughly chopped

1 Preheat the grill to hot.
2 Put all the dressing ingredients in a screw-top jar and shake.
3 Put the onion, courgettes, tomatoes and pepper chunks on a baking sheet and brush with a little dressing. Grill for 8 minutes, until just cooked. Allow to cool slightly, then transfer to a large salad bowl.
4 Add the rocket leaves and the remaining dressing and toss well. Sprinkle over the chopped parsley and serve.

lamb shanks in red wine

serves 4

2 sprigs rosemary,
  leaves finely chopped
2 garlic cloves, crushed
2 tbsp olive oil
4 lamb shanks
600ml/1pt/2½ cups full-bodied red
  wine
1 onion, chopped
2 celery stalks, chopped
2 carrots, chopped
1 handful fresh mint leaves, roughly
  chopped
Freshly ground black pepper

1 Mix the rosemary, garlic and
   oil. Season with pepper.
2 Put the lamb shanks in a
   large, deep dish. Make
   several deep cuts in the meat
   and push a little rosemary
   and garlic mixture into them.
   Spread the remaining mixture over the surface of the
   shanks. Pour over the wine,
   cover and leave in the fridge
   to marinate for at least 2
   hours, preferably overnight.
3 Preheat the oven to
   170°C/325°F/Gas 3. Put the
   onion, celery, carrots and mint
   in an oven-proof dish. Put the
   lamb shanks on top and pour
   over the marinade. Cover and
   cook for 1 hour. Uncover and
   cook for a further hour. Serve.

dessert recipes

hot bananas with pumpkin seeds & lime

serves 4

4 bananas, chopped
1 handful pumpkin seeds
3 tsp desiccated coconut
1 tbsp clear honey (optional)
Freshly squeezed juice of 1 lime
Low-fat fromage frais, to serve

1 Preheat the oven to
   180°C/350°F/Gas 4.
2 Mix all the ingredients except
   the fromage frais in an
   ovenproof dish. Bake for 15
   minutes. Serve warm with the
   fromage frais.

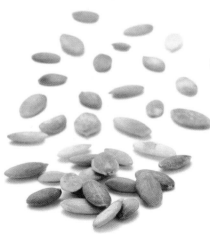

poire au chocolat

serves 4

4 ripe dessert pears
8 walnut halves, chopped
1 handful flaked almonds
1 handful chopped berries, such as
  blueberries or cranberries
100g/3½oz dark chocolate
4 tbsp black decaffeinated coffee,
  cooled
4 tbsp semi-skimmed cow's, almond,
  rice or soy milk

1 Peel the pears and cut a small
   sliver from the base of each so
   it stands upright. Hollow out
   the core from the base of each
   fruit. Leave the top intact.
2 Mix together the nuts and
   berries and press some of this
   mixture into the hollow of each
   pear. Stand the stuffed pears
   upright in a serving dish.
3 Melt the chocolate in a heat-
   proof bowl over a pan of sim-
   mering water. Stir in the coffee
   and milk. Spoon the mixture
   over the pears, then put in the
   fridge for 2–3 hours. Serve with
   the remaining nut and berry
   mixture spooned over the top.

baked peaches
with raspberries

serves 4

4 large peaches
100ml/3½fl oz/1 glass dry white wine
2 handfuls raspberries
Low-fat fromage frais, to serve

1 Preheat the oven to
   180°C/350°F/Gas 4.
2 Put the peaches in a heat-proof
   bowl and cover with boiling
   water. Leave to stand for
   3 minutes. Remove the
   peaches and peel carefully.
   Cut in half and remove the
   stones. Arrange the peach
   halves, cut-side up, in a shallow
   baking dish.
3 Put 4 or 5 raspberries in
   the hollow of each peach
   half, with a little wine.
   Pour the rest of the wine
   around the peaches.
4 Bake for 15–20 minutes. Serve
   warm with the fromage frais.

unsweetened
summer pudding

serves 4

6 thin slices wholemeal bread, crusts
   removed
350g/12oz ripe mixed berries, such as
   strawberries, raspberries,
   blackberries, blueberries and
   redcurrants, washed and hulled
Low-fat fromage frais, to serve

1 Line a small pudding bowl with
   4 slices of the bread – cut them
   into shape so they fit tightly.
   Put the fruit and 2 tablespoons
   of water in a small saucepan
   and gently bring to the boil over
   low heat. Cook for 2 minutes.
2 Spoon the fruit into the

bread-lined bowl, reserving the
excess juice. Cover the fruit
with the remaining slices of
bread. Put a dish on top of the
pudding and a heavy weight on
top of it. Chill in the fridge for
about 8 hours.

3 Remove the weight and the
   dish. Put a serving plate upside-
   down on top of the pudding
   bowl and gently turn them
   over together, so the pudding
   comes out of the bowl onto the
   plate. Pour the reserved juice
   over the pudding. Serve with
   the fromage frais.

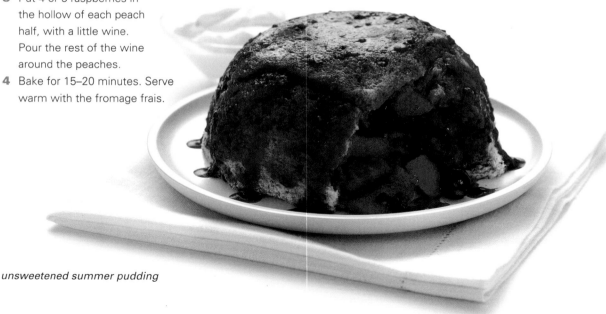

unsweetened summer pudding

the natural health guru programs

bites, snacks and drinks

guacamole

serves 4

1 ripe avocado, peeled and stoned
Freshly squeezed juice of ½ lemon or
  lime
2 tsp extra virgin olive oil
1 small green chilli
Freshly ground black pepper
1 small handful chives, chopped
Wholemeal toast, oatcakes, rice cakes
  or crispbread

1　Put the avocado flesh, lemon
　　or lime juice, oil and chilli in
　　a blender. Whizz to form a
　　smooth paste. Season with
　　black pepper and transfer to a
　　serving bowl. Sprinkle with the
　　chives.
2　Spread the guacamole on the
　　wholemeal toast, oatcakes, rice
　　cakes or crispbread, and serve.

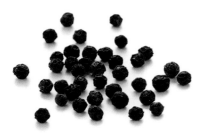

smoked trout and lemon pâté

serves 4

250g/9oz smoked trout fillets
4 tbsp low-fat bio yogurt
Grated zest and freshly squeezed juice
  of 1 unwaxed lemon
1 handful flat-leaf parsley, roughly
  chopped
Freshly ground black pepper
Rye bread, rice cakes or crispbread

1　Flake the trout and remove
　　any bones. Mix in the yogurt,
　　lemon juice and zest and pars-
　　ley. Season with black pepper.
2　Serve on the rye bread, rice
　　cakes or crispbread.

mango and papaya smoothie

serves 4

1 large mango, flesh roughly chopped
1 papaya, flesh roughly chopped
600ml/1pt/2½ cups semi-skimmed
  cow's, almond, rice or soy milk
150ml/5fl oz/½ cup low-fat bio yogurt
1 handful crushed ice

1　Put all the ingredients in a
　　blender and whizz until smooth.
　　Serve immediately.

orange and carrot juice

serves 4

10 large oranges, peeled, pithed and
  quartered
4 large carrots, peeled and chopped
1 handful crushed ice, to serve

1　Whizz the prepared oranges
　　and carrots in a juicer. Serve
　　with the crushed ice.

vegetable stock

makes 3l/6pt

6 carrots, roughly chopped
3 onions, roughly chopped
3 leeks, roughly chopped
3 celery sticks, roughly chopped
1 bunch green leaves, such as lettuce
6 sprigs parsley, including stems
3 sprigs thyme
1 sprig rosemary
1 bay leaf
6 black peppercorns
3.5l/7pt water

1　Put all the ingredients in a large
　　pan, cover and bring to the boil.
　　Skim off any scum. Simmer
　　gently for 1 hour.
2　Cool slightly, then strain. Don't
　　force solids through the sieve
　　unless you want cloudy stock.

introducing the moderate program

The moderate program is more advanced than the gentle program. It's ideal for people who have completed the gentle program and wish to move on; or for those who want greater blood pressure-lowering benefits than those provided by the gentle program. You need to be relatively fit and healthy, and you probably already eat healthily with plenty of fresh fruit and vegetables.

There are 14 daily plans that you can repeat to create a 28-day program. Follow the program for at least a month before assessing its benefits. Once you feel comfortable with the diet and lifestyle changes involved, feel free to make your own adjustments that take into account your tastes and lifestyle.

The moderate program diet

The daily food plans in this program are based on a low-glycemic index (GI) diet. As well as following the principles of the Dietary Approaches to Stop Hypertension (DASH; see page 46), the diet includes more of the superfoods that are particularly beneficial for people with hypertension (see pages 56–59). There are a greater number of vegetarian and fish dishes than in the gentle program, and I also introduce you to home-sprouted beans and seeds, home-made fruit and vegetable juices and a wider variety of grains than you may have eaten previously.

This diet has the potential to lower blood pressure by 7/4 to 11/5mmHg or more within 30 days, even if you are taking anti-hypertensive medications. This style of eating will also lower your total and LDL-cholesterol levels and reduce your triglyceride levels.

As part of the moderate program you may eat a daily 40–50g (approx 1½oz) piece of dark chocolate (at least 70 percent cocoa solids) and drink up to 150ml (5fl oz) red wine per day if you wish. Unsweetened red grape juice provides an alternative source of antioxidants for those who prefer not to drink alcohol.

Sprouting beans and seeds I recommend that you start sprouting your own beans and seeds during the program. You can do this easily in a jam jar, but you can also buy a customized germinator that provides the correct conditions of warmth and humidity for optimal growth. Home-sprouted beans and seeds are a great source of vitamins, minerals, trace elements and live enzymes. You can add them to salads, stir-fries, rice, soups and all kinds of chicken, fish and vegetarian dishes. Simply rinse 4–6 tablespoons of mixed organic beans or seeds in water. Put in a glass jar or sprinkle lightly over a germinator, and allow to germinate for three to five days. Choose any of the following: alfalfa, radish, broccoli, white radish, red clover, mustard and cress seeds; wheat; or lentils, quinoa or mung beans.

Making your own juices I suggest that you invest in a juicer so you can start making your own juices. Freshly prepared juice has a creamy texture, a milky hue and is richer in vitamins and antioxidants than juice that has sat on a shelf or in a fridge for several days. Although you will remove much of the insoluble fibre from the fruit or vegetables when juicing, you obtain significantly more vitamins and minerals than when

Shopping list

You will need all the food and drink items on the shopping list for the gentle program (see page 80). In addition you will need the following (where possible, buy regularly in small quantities for optimum freshness).

drinks
decaffeinated coffee
rosé wine
vanilla rooibos tea

dairy and soy products
firm tofu
silken tofu (soft)

fruit and vegetables
prunes
bean sprouts and seeds for
sprouting
beetroot
black olives (unsalted)
butternut squash
fennel
pomegranate
radicchio
vine leaves
wild mushrooms

nuts and seeds (always
choose unsalted varieties)
cashew nuts
hazelnuts
pine nuts
poppy seeds

herbs and sauces
lemongrass
low-sodium pesto sauce

grains
couscous
hemp pasta
quinoa
red rice
spinach or wholemeal lasgane
sheets
wild rice

proteins
crab
prawns
sea bass
black beans

miscellaneous
rosewater

eating fruit and vegetables in their natural raw state. The secret is in their concentration. One 100ml (3½fl oz) serving of carrot juice can give you as much betacarotene as around 0.5kg (1lb) of raw carrots. Here are some tips for making delicious juices at home:

- Pick garden-fresh fruit and vegetables. As soon as they are harvested, vitamin content drops.
- If possible, buy organic produce that has not come into contact with artificial fertilizers or pesticides.
- Choose firm, plump produce with a good colour.
- Citrus fruit with tough skins need peeling before juicing, but you can process lemons and limes intact for flavour.
- Choose seedless varieties of grape and remove stalks to avoid a bitter taste.
- Some fruits, such as bananas and avocado, can be difficult to juice – they are best mashed or blended and then stirred into other fruit juice bases.
- Virtually any blend of fruit, vegetable or herb is possible – experiment.
- Dilute juice with mineral water for a thirst-quenching drink. Milk can also be added to some juices, such as carrot juice.

Eating a variety of grains Some of the grains in the moderate program may be unfamiliar to you, so here's a brief guide to hemp pasta, red rice, wild rice and quinoa. Hemp pasta is made from flour and oil derived from hemp seeds (related to sunflower seeds). Hemp seeds have a similar protein content to soybeans but are also a rich source of omega-3 oils and vitamin E.

Red rice (such as from the Camargue or Bhutan) has a nutty flavour and a chewy texture. It has the same nutritional value as brown rice but cooks twice as quickly. Wild rice is the seed of a water grass. It's fermented to make it easier to hull and to improve its nutty flavour. It is often mixed with brown or red rice.

Moderate program supplements

The supplements I suggest you take when following the moderate program are similar to those in the gentle program but, where appropriate, at a higher, more therapeutic dose. You can find information about these supplements and their blood-pressure-lowering effects on pages 60–63.

recommended daily supplements

- Vitamin C (1000mg)
- Vitamin E (400i.u/268mg)
- Lycopene carotenoid complex (15mg)
- Selenium (100mcg)
- Co-enzyme Q10 (90mg)
- Garlic tablets (allicin yield 1000mcg–1500mcg)
- Omega-3 fish oil (600mg daily; for example, 2x1g fish oil capsules, each supplying 180mg EPA plus 120mg DHA)

optional daily supplements (these will provide additional health benefits)

- Alpha lipoic acid (200mg). May be combined with L-carnitine in a 1:1 ratio
- Magnesium (300mg)
- Calcium (800mg)
- Folic acid (600mcg) plus vitamin B12 (50mcg)
- Reishi (1000mg)
- Bilberry fruit extracts (120mg – standardized to give 25 percent anthocyanins)
- Probiotics (fermented milk drinks, bio yogurt or supplements)

Quinoa is the seed of a plant related to spinach. It's an excellent source of protein (50 percent higher than most grains), vitamin E and B-group vitamins and folate, as well as minerals such as potassium, magnesium, zinc, copper and manganese.

Foods to avoid or eat less of As I recommend in the gentle program, throw away any foods in your cupboards that are high in sugar, salt, saturated fat and trans fats. Do not be tempted to add salt during cooking or at the table. Obtain flavour from fresh herbs and black pepper instead.

The moderate program exercise routine

The moderate exercise program is designed for those who are relatively fit and who already exercise regularly for 30 minutes on most days of the week. Over the course of the program you will increase the amount of

time you exercise. You will also do weight exercises to complement the aerobic exercise you are taking. In the second half of the program I introduce qigong (see page 44). As well as improving physical well-being, qigong has the power to calm your mind.

When starting an exercise program, always monitor your 10-second pulse rate (see page 69). If you have angina or a history of heart attack, ask your doctor for guidance on how much exercise you can take.

The moderate program therapies

In this program I introduce you to several complementary therapies that can help to reduce your blood pressure. You will find straightforward relaxation techniques to practise on many days of the program. Please look at days seven, thirteen and fourteen of the program now so that you can book appointments with the therapists I advise you to see.

1

the moderate program day one

Daily menu

- Breakfast: home-made muesli (see page 100) with chopped almonds and berries

- Morning snack: a piece of fruit (choose from the selection on the shopping list; see page 80)

- Lunch: half an avocado. Bowl of mixed salad leaves sprinkled with a tablespoon of seeds and balsamic dressing (see page 106). Low-fat bio yogurt with blueberries

- Afternoon snack: a handful of almonds

- Dinner: mushroom and walnut lasagne (see page 139). Broccoli. Baby carrots. 40–50g (about 1½oz) bar dark chocolate

- Drinks: 570ml (1pt) semi-skimmed or skimmed milk. Freshly squeezed fruit/veg juice. Unlimited green/black or white tea, herbal tea and mineral water. 150ml (5fl oz) red wine or unsweetened red grape juice

- Supplements: see page 113

Daily exercise routine

During the first week of this program, I will set muscle-toning exercises that build up into a daily strength and suppleness regime. This is important to prepare you for your slowly increasing level of physical activity. Start with seated leg lifts, which work the muscles in the fronts of your thighs. In addition to the muscle-toning exercises, walk for 30 minutes at a moderate to brisk pace.

Seated leg lifts

1 Sit up straight on the edge of your bed, with your feet flat on the floor and your hands on the bed by your sides.

2 Extend your left leg until it's straight out in front of you.

4 Hold for a count of three, then slowly lower it.

5 Do this 10 times. Repeat with your right leg.

Yoga breathing

Over the next few days I will explain some key yogic breathing techniques, known as pranayama, which you can use to prepare yourself for deeper meditation. Today's technique is known as dirgha – the three-part breath. It is perhaps the most important yogic pranayama because it overcomes the modern affliction of shallow breathing.

Dirgha – the three-part breath

1 Sit comfortably in a cross-legged position, with your back straight. Close your eyes and, as you breathe in and out, focus on the expansion and contraction of your ribcage.

2 Breathe into the lower part of your ribcage and, with each exhalation, allow all tension to flow away.

3 Now breathe into your lower ribcage and then draw more breath in so that the middle part of your ribcage expands.

4 Continue inhaling. Make the third part of your in-breath expand the upper part of your lungs – feel your clavicles (collar bones) rise up.

5 Breathe smoothly in this way for five minutes or as long you want to. If you feel light-headed, stop. End by breathing normally for 10 minutes in quiet contemplation. Carry the sense of calm you have gained into your day.

day two

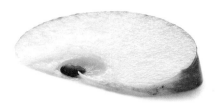

Daily menu

- **Breakfast: porridge with sliced apple**

- **Morning snack: a piece of fruit**

- **Lunch: bowl of sliced green, yellow and red peppers, sprouted beans, celery and mixed salad leaves sprinkled with balsamic dressing (see page 106). Wholemeal or hemp pasta. Low-fat bio yogurt with black or red grapes**

- **Afternoon snack: a handful of walnuts**

- **Dinner: salmon steak baked with lemon, garlic and dill. Steamed green beans drizzled with almond oil. Brown, red or wild rice, or quinoa. Baked banana with low-fat fromage frais**

- **Drinks: 570ml (1pt) semi-skimmed or skimmed milk. Freshly squeezed fruit/veg juice. Unlimited green/black or white tea, herbal tea and mineral water. 150ml (5fl oz) red wine or unsweetened red grape juice**

- **Supplements: see page 113**

Today's dinner-time dessert is baked banana – in Ayurvedic medicine bananas are used to help lower blood pressure. They are a good source of potassium and also have an angiotensin-converting enzyme (ACE) blocking action (highest in ripe bananas).

Daily exercise routine

Walk at a moderate to brisk pace for 30 minutes today. Do your muscle-toning exercise from day one, followed by these seated squats, which tone your arms and legs. To do the squats you will need two small weights of around 450g (1lb) each. These can be either cans of food or dumbbells.

Seated squats

1 Sit on the edge of your bed, so your toes are below your knees and your feet and knees are shoulder-width apart.
2 Hold a weight in each hand, and place your elbows by your sides so the backs of your hands rest lightly on the bed.
3 Take a deep breath in and, as you breathe out, slowly stand up, curling the weights up to your shoulders.

4 Take a deep breath in and, as you breathe out, slowly sit back down while lowering your arms. Do this as slowly as possible, feeling the contraction in your muscles. Repeat 10 times.

Yoga breathing

Today's pranayama can be carried out on almost any occasion, without anyone noticing.

Lengthening your out-breath

1 Sit comfortably, with your arms hanging loosely by your sides. Slowly inhale until your lungs are full of air. Focus on the rise of your abdomen rather than your chest. Breathe out and try to empty your lungs of air.
2 Gradually speed up your inhalations, and slow down your exhalations until you spend 3 seconds breathing in, and 7 seconds breathing out.
3 Keep breathing like this at a rate of just six breaths per minute (half the normal rate). Focus on emptying your lungs, and on keeping air flow continuous – don't hold your breath between inhaling and exhaling. Do this for 5 minutes.

the moderate program day three

Daily menu

- Breakfast: low-fat fromage frais mixed with chopped almonds and blueberries

- Morning snack: piece of fruit

- Lunch: cream of watercress soup (see page 133). Bowl of mixed salad leaves sprinkled with mixed nuts, sprouted beans, dill, grated beetroot and balsamic dressing (see page 106). Oatcakes. Low-fat bio yogurt with black grapes

- Afternoon snack: a handful of almonds

- Dinner: roasted red peppers with herby bulgur wheat (see page 138). Bowl of mixed salad leaves sprinkled with mixed nuts. Tropical fruit salad

- Drinks: 570ml (1pt) semi-skimmed or skimmed milk. Freshly squeezed fruit/veg juice. Unlimited green/black or white tea, herbal tea and mineral water. 150ml (5fl oz) red wine or unsweetened red grape juice

- Supplements: see page 113

As you do your brisk walk today, remind yourself that this one session of moderately intense exercise can lower your blood pressure for up to 24 hours. After three consecutive days of exercise, your blood pressure is reduced for longer. Three out of four people with hypertension show benefits when starting a regular exercise program, with an average blood pressure reduction of 11/8mmHg. Blood pressure returns to pre-exercise levels after one to two weeks of no exercise.

Daily exercise routine

Walk at a moderate to brisk pace for 30 minutes today. Do your muscle-toning exercises from days one and two, followed by the seated bridge, which tones your back, leg and arm muscles.

Seated bridge

1 Sit on the edge of your bed, with your feet flat on the floor and your knees bent at 90 degrees. Rest your palms on the edge of the bed by your sides, fingers facing forward.
2 Take a deep breath in and, as you breathe out, lift your hips

so your weight is supported by your palms and feet. Continue lifting your body and arch your back up until you are in a bridge shape. Hold for 20 seconds (while breathing normally), then slowly sit back down.

Yoga breathing

Today's breathing exercise improves your focus and promotes a sense of power and oneness.

Ujjayi – ocean breath

1 Sit comfortably in a cross-legged position on the floor. Breathe deeply in and out through your mouth. Start to make a soft, whispering, *haaaaahhhh* noise as you breathe out, by slightly constricting the back of your throat – as if you were trying to fog up a window.
2 Do this several times on your out-breath. When you are comfortable doing this, make the same noise as you inhale. Your breathing should sound like the ebb and flow of the ocean.
3 Now practise the same breath but through your nose. Do this for a few minutes.

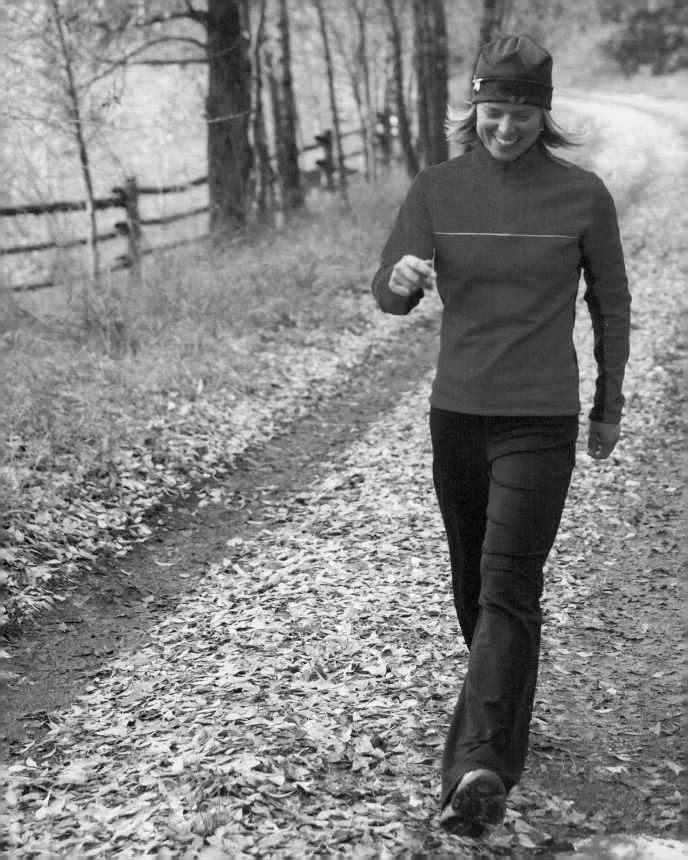

the moderate program day four

Daily menu

- **Breakfast: home-made muesli (see page 100) with dates**

- **Morning snack: a piece of fruit**

- **Lunch: smoked mackerel and mango medley (see page 134). Wholemeal roll. Low-fat bio yogurt with fresh fruit**

- **Afternoon snack: a handful of walnuts**

- **Dinner: stir-fried turkey with bean sprouts (see page 138). Pak choi. Red, brown or wild rice, or quinoa. 40–50g (about 1½oz) bar dark chocolate**

- **Drinks: 570ml (1pt) semi-skimmed or skimmed milk. Freshly squeezed fruit/veg juice. Unlimited green/black or white tea, herbal tea and mineral water. 150ml (5fl oz) red wine or unsweetened red grape juice**

- **Supplements: see page 113**

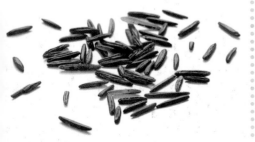

Daily exercise routine

Walk at a moderate to brisk pace for 30 minutes today. Do your muscle-toning exercises from days one to three, followed by this seated triceps dip to tone your upper arms.

Seated triceps dip

1 Sit on the very edge of a bed, with your knees bent and your feet flat on the floor. Place your hands on the edge of the bed, fingers facing forward.

2 Keep your arms straight and lift your bottom off the edge of the bed. Keeping your back straight, and your stomach muscles pulled in, bend your elbows and lower your bottom toward the ground. Make sure your elbows don't pivot outward by slightly squeezing them in toward each other.

3 Straighten your arms to lift your hips again. Repeat five times.

Yoga breathing

Today's breathing exercise teaches you how to interrupt your inhalations. It serves as an introduction to tomorrow's exercise, which lowers blood pressure. You need

only practise today's exercise on this occasion – I have included it so that you can familarize yourself with the technique.

Viloma pranayama stage 1

1 Spend 5 minutes relaxing quietly in corpse pose (see page 97) with your eyes closed.

2 Breathe in for 2 to 3 seconds then hold your breath for 2 to 3 seconds. Breathe in for another 2 to 3 seconds before holding your breath again. Repeat until your lungs are full (normally four to five mini-breaths).

3 Now breathe out slowly and steadily until your lungs feel empty. Breathe normally before repeating the exercise once more. Spend some time resting in quiet contemplation before getting up.

Calming breath

Research shows that yogic breathing promotes reduced oxygen consumption, decreased heart rate and lowered blood pressure.

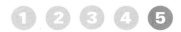

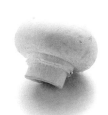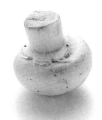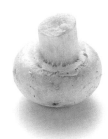

day five

Daily menu

- **Breakfast: spicy garlic mushrooms (see page 132)**

- **Morning snack: a piece of fruit**

- **Lunch: soused herrings (see page 134). Bowl of mixed salad leaves sprinkled with mixed seeds and walnut oil. Wholemeal roll. Low-fat bio yogurt. Kiwi fruit**

- **Afternoon snack: a handful of almonds**

- **Dinner: cinnamon aubergines (see page 136). Spinach. Sweetcorn. Wholemeal or hemp pasta. Oatmeal flummery (see page 140)**

- **Drinks: 570ml (1pt) semi-skimmed or skimmed milk. Freshly squeezed fruit/veg juice. Unlimited green/black or white tea, herbal tea and mineral water. 150ml (5fl oz) red wine or unsweetened red grape juice**

- **Supplements: see page 113**

Today's main meal contains aubergine, a vegetable that is believed to help reduce cholesterol levels partly through antioxidant action, and partly by stimulating bile production in the liver so that more cholesterol is excreted. Although recipes often suggest drawing out the bitter juices from aubergine using salt, I don't advise this. Salting is highly unsuitable for anyone with hypertension; and the bitter ingredients give aubergine its important health benefits.

Daily exercise routine

Walk at a moderate to brisk pace for 30 minutes today. Do your muscle-toning exercises from days one to four, followed by kneeling leg lifts, which tone your buttocks and the backs of your thighs.

Kneeling leg lifts

1 Kneel on all fours with your head slightly down, and your back straight and parallel to the floor.
2 Extend one leg back so it's completely straight behind you. Hold for a count of three, then return to kneeling on all fours.
3 Do 10 of these with each leg.

Yoga breathing

Viloma pranayama stage 2 is an advanced breathing exercise that is used to reduce hypertension. Its rhythm is easier to understand once you have tried yesterday's interrupted breathing exercise.

Viloma pranayama stage 2

1 Spend 5 minutes resting quietly in corpse pose (see page 97) with your eyes closed.
2 When you feel ready, exhale completely until your lungs feel empty. Then inhale smoothly until your lungs feel full.
3 Exhale slowly for 2 or 3 seconds, then pause, holding your breath for 2 to 3 seconds. Exhale further for 2 to 3 seconds before pausing again. Repeat until your lungs feel empty (usually four to five pauses).
4 Breathe in and out normally a few times, then repeat.
5 Do between five and 10 interrupted exhalations. With practice, you can spend 10 minutes alternating interrupted exhalations with three cycles of normal breathing. To finish, lie quietly, breathing normally.

the moderate program day six

Daily menu

- **Breakfast: home-made muesli (see page 100) with added almonds, linseeds and berries**

- **Morning snack: a piece of fruit**

- **Lunch: chickpea and avocado hummus (see page 141). Oatcakes. Bowl of mixed salad leaves sprinkled with mixed seeds, sprouted beans and balsamic dressing (see page 106). Low-fat bio yogurt with fresh fruit**

- **Afternoon snack: a handful of walnuts**

- **Dinner: roast tomato and red pepper soup (see page 135). Grilled, skinless chicken breasts marinated in olive oil and lime juice. Broccoli. Red, brown or wild rice, or quinoa**

- **Drinks: 570ml (1pt) semi-skimmed or skimmed milk. Freshly squeezed fruit/veg juice. Unlimited green/black or white tea, herbal tea and mineral water. 150ml (5fl oz) red wine or unsweetened red grape juice**

- **Supplements: see page 113**

Removing the skin from chicken and other poultry makes your meal more healthy. Tonight's meal would contain 17g (³/₅oz) fat per 100g (3½oz) with the skin on the chicken breast, but only 2.2g (²/₂₅oz) per 100g (3½oz) without the skin.

Daily exercise routine

Having walked every day this week, I suggest you now start a cycling regime. Ideally, cycle every other day, and walk on those days when you are not cycling. You can cycle outdoors (wear a helmet) or on a fixed exercise bike. Do your muscle-toning exercises from days one to five, followed by kneeling leg raises that work on your upper thighs and buttocks.

Kneeling leg raises

1 Kneel on all fours with your head slightly down, and your back parallel to the floor.
2 Extend your right leg straight out behind you. Bend your right knee to 90 degrees, so the sole of your foot is parallel to the ceiling. Using small movements, lift your right foot up and down 10 times.

3 Lower your leg back down to the starting position. Repeat the exercise three times. Repeat with your left leg.

Yoga breathing

Today's technique promotes quietness and is used therapeutically for people with hypertension.

Alternate nostril breathing

1 Sit comfortably with your back straight (cross-legged on the floor is ideal).
2 When you feel ready, close your right nostril with your thumb. Breathe in through your left nostril, slowly and deeply while counting to four.
3 Release your right nostril and use your ring and little fingers to close your left nostril. Now breathe out through your right nostril while counting to eight.
4 Breathe in through the right nostril to a count of four.
5 Release the left nostril, close the right nostril with your thumb and exhale through the left nostril to a count of eight. Do this cycle twice at first. Work up to 10 repetitions. End with quiet contemplation.

day seven

Daily menu

- **Breakfast: vanilla rooibos compote (see page 132). Low-fat bio yogurt**

- **Morning snack: a piece of fruit**

- **Lunch: cream of watercress soup (see page 133). Bowl of mixed salad leaves sprinkled with mixed seeds, bean sprouts, grated beetroot, chopped mint and balsamic dressing (see page 106). Wholemeal roll or pitta bread. Low-fat bio yogurt with fresh fruit**

- **Afternoon snack: a handful of almonds**

- **Dinner: mushroom and walnut lasagne (see page 139). Spinach. Baby carrots. Creamy Turkish delight figs (see page 140)**

- **Drinks: 570ml (1pt) semi-skimmed or skimmed milk. Freshly squeezed fruit/veg juice. Unlimited green/black or white tea, herbal tea and mineral water. 150ml (5fl oz) red wine or unsweetened red grape juice**

- **Supplements: see page 113**

Daily exercise routine

Go for a brisk 35-minute walk today. Do your muscle-toning exercises from days one to six, followed by plank raises, which tone your arms and abdominals.

Plank raises

1 Lie face down on the floor with your arms bent and hands flat on the floor near your shoulders ready to do a press-up. Press your toes into the ground, pull in your abdominal muscles and straighten your arms to lift your body into a straight, plank-like line from your heels to your head.

2 Stay in the plank position for 3 seconds, then slowly lower yourself to the ground. Do this five times.

Consulting a medical herbalist

Now this first week is over, I suggest that you visit a medical herbalist who will select the herbal remedies that are most likely to suit you as an individual. In the first consultation, which usually lasts one hour, a herbalist will assess your general health and ask about any medicines and supplements you are taking. He or she will ask you about your diet, work, life-style, medical history and current physical, mental and emotional state. A herbalist will examine your pulse and may listen to your heart and lungs. He or she will give you one or more herbal remedies to take away. Herbs are often prescribed as tinctures (made by steeping herbs in alcohol) or as decoctions (in which herbs are boiled in water). Herbal tablets and capsules are also used. The results of treatment are assessed in 15–30-minute follow-ups. As a guide, expect to need a month of treatment for every year that you have had hypertension. To find a herbalist, see page 174.

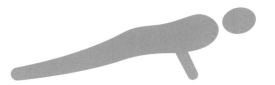

the moderate program day eight

Daily menu

- **Breakfast: banana cinnamon porridge (see page 100)**

- **Morning snack: a piece of fruit**

- **Lunch: bowl of chopped avo-cado and tomatoes mixed with sprouted beans, pomegranate and radicchio in a balsamic dressing (see page 106). Wholemeal roll. Low-fat bio yogurt with fresh fruit**

- **Afternoon snack: a handful of walnuts**

- **Dinner: mock caviar (see page 141). Salmon steak marinated in olive oil and lime juice and baked. Red, brown or wild rice, or qui-noa. Spinach with olive oil**

- **Drinks: 570ml (1pt) semi-skimmed or skimmed milk. Freshly squeezed fruit/veg juice. Unlimited green/black or white tea, herbal tea and mineral water. 150ml (5fl oz) red wine or unsweetened red grape juice**

- **Supplements: see page 113**

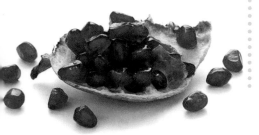

Daily exercise routine

Go for a brisk 35-minute walk today, or cycle for 20 minutes. Do your muscle-toning exercises from days one to seven. Today, I introduce a sequence of qigong exercises (see page 44) that will help you wind down at the end of the day. The opening position will prepare your mind and body for the sequence. Return to this posture between each qigong exercise.

Qigong opening position

1 Stand straight with your feet close together and touching, toes pointing forward. Let your arms relax at your sides with your palms facing inward. Unlock your knees.

2 Relax your body – imagine you are a puppet on a string. Keep your head up, looking forward. Part your lips and lightly touch the roof of your mouth with the tip of your tongue. Breathe gently in through your nose and out through your mouth.

Meditation

From today onward, spend 15 minutes a day in quiet meditation/ visualization – this is a powerful tool that can significantly reduce your blood pressure. Here is the first meditation.

The inner smile

1 Sit or stand comfortably and practise one of the breathing techniques you have learned. Now imagine something that makes you smile. Allow the smile to shine out of your eyes and travel inward.

2 Focus on your navel area. Let the smile radiate here. Become relaxed and calm. See if you can feel a warmth or vibration in the pit of your stomach.

Music therapy

Research shows that classical music can relax you, which is good for your blood pres-sure. In a study, one group of people listened to Mozart, another group listened to new age music, and a third group read magazines. After three days, those listening to Mozart reported the highest levels of peacefulness, mental quiet and relaxation.

day nine

Daily menu

- **Breakfast: figs with pomegranate (see page 132)**

- **Morning snack: a piece of fruit**

- **Lunch: black bean compote with cumin and coriander (see page 133). Bowl of mixed salad leaves sprinkled with mixed seeds and drizzled with walnut oil. Wholemeal roll. Low-fat bio yogurt with fruit**

- **Afternoon snack: toasted mixed nuts (see page 141)**

- **Dinner: stuffed vine leaves with tzatziki (see page 136). Bowl of mixed salad leaves sprinkled with black olives and mixed seeds in a balsamic dressing (see page 106). Mulled fruit salad (see page 140)**

- **Drinks: 570ml (1pt) semi-skimmed or skimmed milk. Freshly squeezed fruit/veg juice. Unlimited green/black or white tea, herbal tea and mineral water. 150ml (5fl oz) red wine or unsweetened red grape juice**

- **Supplements: see page 113**

Daily exercise routine

Go for a brisk 35-minute walk today, or cycle for 20 minutes. Do your muscle-toning exercises from days one to seven. In the evening practise the qigong posture from day eight, and then do the following exercise, which opens the heart and lungs and encourages the free flow of qi.

Qigong – opening the heart

1. In the opening position, breathe in and raise your arms in front of you to shoulder height. As you breathe out, make a breast-stroke movement: extend your arms to the sides, bend your elbows and bring your hands together in front of your chest.
2. Continue this movement for 1 minute. Then stand in contemplation for 1 minute.

Visualization

This powerful visualization will help to lower your blood pressure.

Blue light visualization

1. Sit quietly with your eyes closed. Imagine your body as a pulsating, red shape.
2. Imagine a light bulb is switched on above you. It gives out healing blue light that bathes your body and enters your cells.
3. Visualize your pulsating red shape change to a gentle, undulating blue form. Bask in the cool, restful glow as the blue light lowers your blood pressure. Relax in the light for 15 minutes.

Stress-busting

Stress makes hypertension worse, so it's important to pinpoint the causes of stress and tackle them. Common causes are relationship or work problems or feeling that there is "never enough time". Try to learn time management skills, and how to prioritize tasks and delegate. Pace yourself – make time for exercise and meals. Take regular breaks. Try to separate work from home and learn how to be assertive so that you are effective at expressing your needs. If self-help techniques don't work, consider going on a stress-management course or seeing a stress counsellor.

the moderate program day ten

Daily menu

- **Breakfast: home-made muesli (see page 100)**

- **Morning snack: a piece of fruit**

- **Lunch: warm chickpea salad (see page 134). Bowl of mixed salad leaves sprinkled with mixed nuts, grated beetroot and extra virgin olive oil. Low-fat bio yogurt with fresh fruit**

- **Afternoon snack: a handful of walnuts**

- **Dinner: rosé trout (see page 139). Purple-sprouting broccoli. Sweet potatoes. Sweetcorn. Oatmeal flummery (see page 140)**

- **Drinks: 570ml (1pt) semi-skimmed or skimmed milk. Freshly squeezed fruit/veg juice. Unlimited green/black or white tea, herbal tea and mineral water. 150ml (5fl oz) red wine or unsweetened red grape juice**

- **Supplements: see page 113**

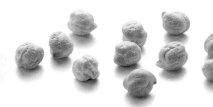

Today's dinner is trout cooked in rosé wine; trout contains a useful amount of omega-3 fatty acids, while the addition of almonds and wine increases the antioxidant value and cholesterol-lowering properties of this tasty dish.

Daily exercise routine

Go for a brisk 35-minute walk today, or cycle for 20 minutes. Do your muscle-toning exercises from days one to seven. In the evening, practise the qigong exercises from days eight and nine, and then do the following exercise.

Qigong – directing qi internally

1. Stand in the opening position. Rub your hands together then place your hands on the base of your ribcage – your right hand on the right side and your left hand on the left. Move your hands in a circle and visualize qi flowing from your hands into your liver on the right, and your spleen on the left.

2. Feel the heat welling up in your hands and travelling into your body, helping your internal organs to function.

3. Move your hands over your

sternum and navel. Visualize qi passing from your hands into your heart and major blood vessels. Finally, move your palms to your lower back and visualize qi flowing into your kidneys and adrenal glands.

4. Continue for as long as you feel qi flowing strongly, then return to the opening position.

Acupressure

This acupressure technique will help you relax. Find your third eye point – between your eyebrows on the bridge of your nose. Massage this point firmly with your dominant middle finger. Make small rotating movements over the point, both clockwise and anti-clockwise, to reduce an excess of stagnant qi. Manipulate this point for 3 minutes to help clear and calm your mind.

Bike power
As you get fitter, you can slowly increase the intensity of your cycling by pedalling faster or riding up hills.

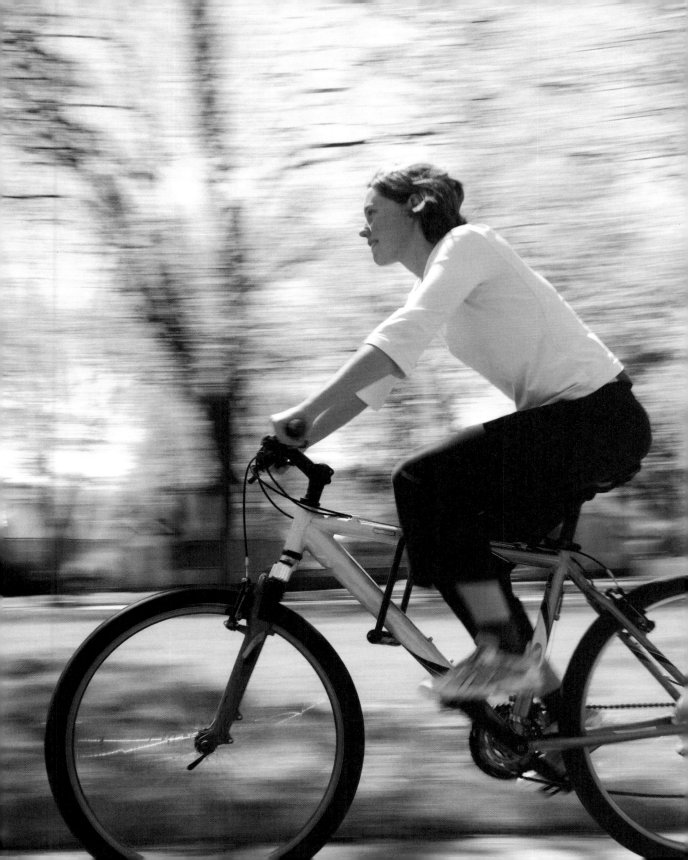

the moderate program day eleven

Daily menu

- **Breakfast: raspberry and Brazil nut medley (see page 133)**

- **Morning snack: a piece of fruit**

- **Lunch: cream of watercress soup (see page 133). Wholemeal roll. Low-fat bio yogurt with fresh fruit**

- **Afternoon snack: berry smoothie (see page 141)**

- **Dinner: grilled mushrooms with almonds and basil (see page 140). Roasted vegetables (baby vine tomatoes, courgettes, aubergine, red pepper and red onion). Wholemeal or hemp pasta. 40–50g (about 1½oz) bar dark chocolate**

- **Drinks: 570ml (1pt) semi-skimmed or skimmed milk. Freshly squeezed fruit/veg juice. Unlimited green/black or white tea, herbal tea and mineral water. 150ml (5fl oz) red wine or unsweetened red grape juice**

- **Supplements: see page 113**

Daily exercise routine

Go for a brisk 40-minute walk today, or cycle for 25 minutes. Do your muscle-toning exercises from days one to seven. In the evening, practise the qigong exercises from days eight to ten, and then do the following exercise, which directs qi down through your body to promote a sense of calm and improve your circulation.

Qigong – directing qi downward

1 Stand in the opening position. Breathe in deeply. Raise your arms and bring your palms together in a prayer-like gesture in front of your upper chest.
2 Carefully raise your left leg and bend it so your left ankle rests on your right knee. As you breathe out, gently bend your right leg and let your weight sink into it. Maintain your balance here for 30–60 seconds. Repeat with the other leg. Return to the opening position for quiet contemplation.

Muscle relaxation

Close the curtains, light some candles and play some classical music for this relaxation exercise.

Progressive muscle relaxation 1

1 Lie down on a mat or bed, close your eyes and breathe slowly and deeply. Begin by clenching your toes. Hold for a count of 10, then relax. Feel the tension drop away.
2 Flex your feet. Hold for a count of 10 then release and let all the tension go.
3 Move slowly up your body, through your legs, buttocks, abdomen, back, shoulders, arms, hands, fingers, neck and head, clenching then relaxing each group of muscles.
4 Keep checking back on the muscles you have worked on to ensure tension has not crept back into them. Once your whole body is relaxed, lie quietly for 10 minutes.

Tension scan
At various points in your day, stop and mentally scan your body for areas of muscle tension. Are muscles in your back, shoulder or jaw carrying tension? If so, make a point of releasing that tension.

day twelve

Daily menu

- **Breakfast: spicy garlic mushrooms (see page 132)**

- **Morning snack: a piece of fruit**

- **Lunch: bowl of mixed salad leaves sprinkled with mixed seeds, grated beetroot and walnut oil. Wholemeal pitta bread or granary roll. Low-fat bio yogurt with fresh fruit**

- **Afternoon snack: a handful of walnuts**

- **Dinner: French onion soup (see page 135). Skinless chicken or turkey piece, marinated in olive oil and fresh herbs, then grilled. Spinach. Couscous**

- **Drinks: 570ml (1pt) semi-skimmed or skimmed milk. Freshly squeezed fruit/veg juice. Unlimited green/black or white tea, herbal tea and mineral water. 150ml (5fl oz) red wine or unsweetened red grape juice**

- **Supplements: see page 113**

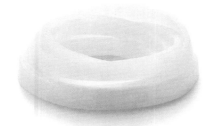

Today's French onion soup is a delicious and nutritious start to your dinner. Onions contain similar sulphur-containing phytochemicals to garlic (see page 57).

Daily exercise routine

Go for a brisk 40-minute walk today, or cycle for 25 minutes. Do your muscle-toning exercises from days one to seven. In the evening, wind down with the qigong sequence from days eight to eleven, and then do the following.

Qigong – balancing blood pressure

1 Stand in the opening position. Stretch your right arm out to the side so it's parallel to the floor, palm facing upward. Now arch your left arm up to form a gentle curve, with your palm facing the top of your head.

2 Move your weight onto your left leg, bending it slightly at the knee. Keep your right leg straight and raise your right heel slightly off the ground. Turn your head to look at your right hand.

3 Now arch your right arm overhead and stretch your left arm

out to the side, palm facing up. At the same time, move your weight onto your right leg, bending slightly at the knee. Straighten your left leg and let your left heel rise slightly. Turn to look to the left.

4 Move gently from side to side in this way, several times.

Relaxation

Today's technique is similar to yesterday's, but promotes a deeper level of muscle awareness.

Progressive muscle relaxation 2

1 Lie down, close your eyes and breathe deeply. Bend your toes slightly so just a little tension enters them. Count to 10, then relax – feel tension drop away.

2 Flex your feet slightly. Hold for a count of 10 then release – feel the tension go.

3 Work your way up your body minimally tightening each group of muscles then relaxing them. Be aware of how a slightly tensed muscle feels different from a fully relaxed muscle.

4 Finish by minimally tensing every muscle in your body at the same time, then let go.

the moderate program day thirteen

Daily menu

- **Breakfast: figs with pomegranate (see page 132)**

- **Morning snack: a piece of fruit**

- **Lunch: smoked mackerel and mango medley (see page 134). Bowl of mixed salad leaves sprinkled with sprouting beans, grated beetroot and fennel, mixed seeds and walnut oil. Low-fat bio yogurt**

- **Afternoon snack: a handful of almonds**

- **Dinner: stir-fried bean sprouts, carrots, spring onions, mushrooms, sugarsnap peas and broccoli, with ginger, garlic, coriander and lemongrass. Red, brown or wild rice, or quinoa. Stewed, unsweetened rhubarb with low-fat vanilla fromage frais**

- **Drinks: 570ml (1pt) semi-skimmed or skimmed milk. Freshly squeezed fruit/veg juice. Unlimited green/black or white tea, herbal tea and mineral water. 150ml (5fl oz) red wine or unsweetened red grape juice**

- **Supplements: see page 113**

Daily exercise routine

Go for a brisk 40-minute walk or cycle for 25 minutes today. Do your muscle-toning exercises from days one to seven. In the evening, wind down with the qigong sequence from days eight to twelve, and then add the following exercise, which involves a visualization to remove stagnant qi and replenish it with fresh, universal qi.

Qigong – removing stagnant qi

1 Stand in the opening position. Breathe in deeply and raise your arms above your head.
2 As you breathe out, lower your arms and visualize stagnant qi being drawn out of your body, through the soles of your feet, deep into the earth. As it drains away, imagine fresh qi coming in through the top of your head. Feel tension and fatigue drain away as your qi is recharged.
3 Visualize the fresh qi flowing through your body, then settling just below your navel (in an area called the tan tien; see page 44). With practice, you may start to feel a vibration and warmth in this area as qi becomes concentrated there.

Floatation therapy

Today, I'd like you to book a series of at least four floatations at your nearest float centre. Floatation therapy can help you achieve the deepest relaxation possible without falling asleep, and a single float lasting 45 minutes has been shown to lower hypertension. You lie in a light-proof, sound-insulated tank containing a shallow pool of water at skin temperature, to which Epsom salts (magnesium sulphate) is added. This forms a super-saturated solution of saline that is even more buoyant than the Dead Sea. Floating frees your brain from its usual sensory distractions; as a result, your brain more easily generates theta waves, which are associated with feelings of calm.

Plant therapy
Looking at green plants helps to reduce blood pressure and anxiety during stressful activities. Relaxing in a room with a view of a tree produces a more rapid reduction in blood pressure than relaxing in a viewless room.

day fourteen

Daily menu

- **Breakfast: home-made muesli (see page 100) with pomegranate and blueberries**

- **Morning snack: a piece of fruit**

- **Lunch: baked sweet potato. Low-fat cottage cheese. Rocket. Bean sprouts with grated beet-root, celery and walnuts. Low-fat bio yogurt with fresh fruit**

- **Afternoon snack: a handful of walnuts**

- **Dinner: sea bass with lime and coriander (see page 135). Broccoli. Couscous. Walnut and fruit compote (see page 140)**

- **Drinks: 570ml (1pt) semi-skimmed or skimmed milk. Freshly squeezed fruit/veg juice. Unlimited green/black or white tea, herbal tea and mineral water. 150ml (5fl oz) red wine or unsweetened red grape juice**

- **Supplements: see page 113**

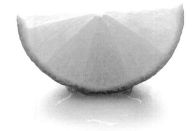

Daily exercise routine

Today, and from now on, walk briskly for 45 minutes or cycle for 30 minutes on most days of the week. Also do your muscle-toning exercises from days one to seven. In the evening, wind down with the qigong sequence. Today's exercise, in which you redirect qi to the tan tien, completes the sequence.

Qigong – closing exercise

1 Stand in the opening position. Let your body sink a little at your knees and waist, then bring your hands to the front of your body, at the level of your navel, palms facing upward and the tips of your fingers almost touching.
2 Breathe in and raise qi by straightening your body and gently curving your arms up until your palms face your forehead.
3 Breathe out and turn your palms downward – push them down as far as they will go, then let your arms relax.
4 Repeat this raising and lower-ing six times. Then bring your hands to rest on top of each

other over your tan tien. Visualize qi energy flowing out of your hands into your navel area. After a minute or two, return to the opening position.

Consulting a reflexologist

Today, I suggest a consultation with a reflexologist. Reflexology works on reflex points on your feet. Having asked you about your medical history as well as your current health and lifestyle, a reflexologist will ask you to remove your footwear and relax on a seat or couch with your feet raised. He or she will apply a light dusting of talcum powder to their hands, then use their fingers and thumbs to stimulate reflex points all over your feet. The aim is to find any points of tenderness and then massage these points to break up deposits under the skin. This promotes energy flow and opens up blocked nerve pathways. Your treatment will then focus on areas of the foot associated with high blood pressure (see page 38). A session usually lasts 45–60 minutes. Afterwards, you will feel a profound sense of relaxation. To find a reflexologist, see page 175.

continuing the moderate program

Well done! You have followed the moderate program for two weeks. Now I would like you to continue with the eating plan for two more weeks. This will give you an entire month of healthy eating and make you very well-acquainted with the foods you need to buy and eat. After this point you can start to vary the foods you eat, and include some new recipes. The following information will enable you to plan your long-term future using the moderate program principles.

Your long-term diet

The diet you have been following is an advanced, lower glycemic index diet that, as well as following the basic principles of the DASH diet (see page 46), also includes extra foods that are beneficial for people with hypertension. These superfoods (see pages 56–59) have a significant blood pressure-lowering effect. These guidelines will help you continue on this diet:

- Include as many superfoods, such as almonds, apples, oats, oily fish and pumpkin seeds, as you can every day (see pages 56–59 for a complete list).
- Continue to use the low-glycemic index grains included in the moderate plan, such as hemp pasta, red rice, wild rice and quinoa.
- Every week, have two or three vegetarian days, eat fish two or three times, and meat only once or twice.
- Sprout a variety of beans and seeds at home.
- Keep making your own combinations of fruit and vegetable juices, and fresh herbal teas.

Recipes Explore fish-based and vegetarian recipes – you will find some at www.naturalhealthguru.co.uk and you can post your favourites there, too, for other followers of the moderate program to try. You don't have to follow formal recipes on the moderate program: simply grilling or baking fish with olive oil, lemon/lime juice, fresh herbs and black pepper provides a delicious, quick and healthy meal. Team this with lightly steamed fresh vegetables or a salad, plus a low-glycemic index grain, and you have a meal that is beneficial to the health of your cardiovascular system.

Selecting fish Because fish will play a prominent part in your long-term diet it's useful to know how to select fish that is in optimum condition – and also how much to buy. Here are some guidelines:

- Try to buy fish directly from a fishmonger or fishermen's co-operative.
- Inspect the fish – its skin should gleam like finest shot silk. It should smell of seawater – salty, with a tang of ozone, rather than smelling fishy. A fishy smell is the result of chemical breakdown that suggests the fish is not optimally fresh. The eyes of the fish should be clear, bright and shiny, the gills should be a healthy pink or bright red and the scales should be tight.
- Perform the "prod test" – poke the flesh with your finger. It should feel moist and firm to the touch, and spring back with elasticity, rather than remain collapsed. This test is useful even if the fish is

ultra-fresh – even fresh fish can be flabby and in poor condition.

- Pick up shellfish to assess their weight – they should always seem heavy for their size. Make sure bivalve molluscs such as mussels shut firmly on tapping and are not coated with decaying weeds, barnacles or mud.
- Wastage with fish varies from around one-third with monkfish to more than two-thirds with lobster. As a general rule, buy double or triple the amount you want to eat. Don't discard bones – boil them up with herbs and vegetables to make fish stock.

Your long-term supplement regime

Continue taking the recommended supplements for the moderate program (see page 113) long term. If you have taken only the supplements on the recommended list, you may wish to add in one or more of the supplements in the optional list for extra benefit. Full details of each supplement, including updates on latest research findings, are available at www.naturalhealth-guru.co.uk

Your exercise routine

After two weeks of doing the muscle-toning exercises, you should have started to notice a difference in your muscle tone. Continue these exercises and, if you do not yet belong to a gym, consider joining one and having a session with a personal trainer. Aim to do at least 45 minutes of aerobic exercise on most days, and continue the qigong exercises at the end of the day.

Your therapy program

Continue to meditate at least once a day for 20 minutes, or, ideally, once in the morning and once in the evening. Also continue doing any of the breathing exercises as these can intensify the power of your meditation. If you find it helpful, visit a medical

Sleep quality
Pay attention to the quality of your sleep. Poor sleep is both a source of and a cause of stress. Follow these basic sleep guidelines: go to bed at the same time each night; avoid anything that is stimulating or stressful in the evenings (for example, caffeine, a large meal, exercise or work); make sure your bedroom is dark and peaceful; and get sufficient exercise and natural light during the day.

herbalist and/or a reflexologist on a regular basis. Consider booking regular float sessions at a floatation centre if you found the experience relaxing.

Monitoring your blood pressure

While continuing with the moderate program, monitor your blood pressure on a weekly basis, at the same time of day, unless your doctor has asked you to check it more frequently. Record your blood pressure measurements in a chart (use a copy of the one on page 77), so you have an easily accessible record.

If your blood pressure is consistently below 130/80mmHg, well done. The moderate program suits you and you should continue it long term. If you are taking anti-hypertensive medication, your doctor may consider reducing this, if he or she judges that it's appropriate. This is not something you should do without your doctor's supervision as certain anti-hypertensive drugs need to be reduced slowly.

If your blood pressure is consistently between 130/80mmHg and 140/90mmHg, consider moving up to the full-strength program to see if you can bring it down to below 130/80mmHg.

If your blood pressure is consistently above 140/90mmHg, you can move onto the full-strength program, but you should also consult your doctor.

breakfast recipes

vanilla rooibos compote

. . . .

serves 4

1 vanilla rooibos herbal teabag
300ml/½pt/1 cup boiling water
8 slices dried apple
8 dried apricots
8 dried figs
8 dried prunes
1 handful raisins
Low-fat fromage frais or bio yogurt, to serve
1 handful flaked almonds, walnut halves or mixed seeds, to serve (optional)

1 Put the teabag in a heat-proof bowl, pour over the water and leave until cool. Remove the teabag.
2 Put the dried fruit in a bowl, pour over the tea and leave in the fridge overnight. Top each serving with fromage frais or yogurt, and nuts or seeds.

spicy garlic mushrooms

. . . .

serves 4

2 shallots, sliced
2 spring onions, sliced
5cm/2in piece fresh ginger, peeled and grated
2 garlic cloves, crushed
1 red chilli, deseeded and sliced
450g/1lb button mushrooms, halved
1 tbsp olive oil
150ml/5fl oz/1⅓glasses dry white wine
1 handful fresh coriander or flat-leaf parsley, roughly chopped
4 slices wholemeal toast, to serve
Freshly ground black pepper

1 Fry the shallots, spring onions, ginger, garlic, chilli and mushrooms in the oil.
2 Add the white wine and simmer gently. Season and stir in the herbs. Serve hot on toast.

figs with pomegranate

. . . .

serves 4

1 pomegranate
8 fresh figs
125ml/4fl oz/½ cup low-fat fromage frais

1 Slice the crown end off the pomegranate and score the rind from top to bottom, in six places around the fruit. Put the pomegranate in a bowl of water and break the sections apart. Tear away the thin membranes and pry out the seeds. The seeds will sink, while the bitter-tasting membranes and skin will float for easy separation. Drain, reserving the seeds.
2 Make 2 deep cuts in the top of each fig to form a cross. Gently open out the figs, so that each one forms a tulip-like shape Mix the fromage frais with the pomegranate seeds, saving a few seeds to serve.
3 Put the figs on a serving plate. Spoon the fromage frais mixture into the figs, and serve any remaining on the side. Sprinkle with the reserved pomegranate seeds and serve.

figs with pomegranate

lunch recipes

raspberry and brazil nut medley

serves 4

400g/14oz raspberries
300g/10½oz silken tofu, roughly cut into chunks
100g/3½oz/²/₃ cup Brazil nuts, roughly chopped

1 Set 2 tablespoons of raspberries aside for serving. Put the remaining raspberries in a blender with the tofu and process until smooth. Divide the mixture between 4 glass serving bowls.
2 Sprinkle the chopped Brazil nuts over each serving, top with the reserved raspberries and serve.

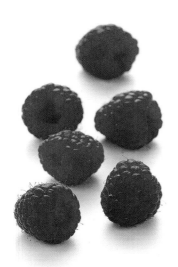

black bean compote with cumin and coriander

serves 4

250g/9oz/1¼ cups dried black beans, soaked overnight
½ tbsp extra virgin olive oil
1 large red onion, chopped
1 large green pepper, chopped
2 garlic cloves, crushed
1 tsp cumin seeds, freshly ground
4 medium tomatoes, skinned, deseeded and chopped
1 handful fresh coriander leaves, roughly chopped
Freshly squeezed juice of 1 lime
Freshly ground black pepper
Crusty wholemeal bread, to serve

1 Drain and rinse the beans, put in a pan, cover with water and bring to the boil. Simmer gently for 1–1½ hours until tender. Drain and set aside.
2 Heat the oil in a pan. Add the onion, green pepper, garlic and cumin, and stir-fry for 5 minutes. Add the tomatoes and beans and almost cover with cold water. Bring to the boil, then simmer for 10 minutes.
3 Stir in the coriander leaves and lime juice. Season with black pepper and serve with bread.

cream of watercress soup

serves 4

2 medium potatoes, peeled and roughly chopped
1 onion, chopped
2 garlic cloves, crushed
1l/35fl oz/4 cups vegetable stock (see page 109) or water
1 large bunch watercress, roughly chopped
150ml/5fl oz/²/₃ cup low-fat fromage frais
Freshly grated nutmeg
Freshly ground black pepper

1 Put the potatoes, onion, garlic and stock in a large saucepan. Bring to the boil, lower the heat and leave to simmer gently for 15 minutes.
2 Add the watercress to the pan and cook for a further 5 minutes. Allow to cool slightly, then purée in a blender, in batches if necessary. Stir in the fromage frais, then season to taste with nutmeg or black pepper. Serve hot or cold.

warm chickpea salad

serves 4

½ tbsp extra virgin olive oil
1 red onion, chopped
2 cloves garlic, crushed
1 red pepper, roughly chopped
400g/14oz tin chickpeas, drained
1 large tomato, skinned, deseeded and chopped
Freshly squeezed juice of 1 lemon
1 handful bean sprouts
1 handful fresh parsley or dill, roughly chopped
Freshly ground black pepper
Wholemeal pitta bread, to serve

1 Heat the oil in a large pan. Add the onion, garlic and red pepper and cook over medium heat until soft. Stir in the chickpeas and cook until hot and starting to colour.

2 Add the tomato and lemon juice and cook for 2 minutes. Add the bean sprouts and stir over gentle heat, until warm. Stir in the parsley or dill and season with black pepper. Serve with warmed pitta bread.

smoked mackerel and mango medley

serves 4

250g/9oz mixed baby salad leaves
4 peppered, smoked mackerel fillets, skinned and chopped into bite-sized pieces
1 large, ripe mango, peeled, stoned and flesh cubed
1 ripe avocado, peeled, stoned and flesh cubed
4 spring onions, chopped
1 handful bean sprouts
1 handful fresh coriander leaves
Freshly squeezed juice of 1 lime
2 tbsp extra virgin olive oil or walnut oil
1 tsp clear honey

1 Put the salad leaves in a serving bowl. Carefully mix together the mackerel, mango, avocado, spring onions, bean sprouts and coriander leaves in another bowl and set aside.

2 Put the lime juice, oil and honey in a screw-top jar and shake vigorously. Pour over the mackerel and mango mixture and toss to mix through. Tip the mackerel mixture over the salad leaves and serve.

soused herrings

serves 4

For the marinade:
300ml/10½fl oz/1 cup red wine vinegar
2 juniper berries
2 cloves
1 bay leaf
3 black peppercorns, crushed

4 large herrings, gutted and cleaned with heads and backbones removed
4 tsp wholegrain mustard
4 shallots, thinly sliced
Rye bread, to serve

1 Preheat the oven to 180°C/350°F/Gas 4.

2 Put the marinade ingredients in a pan and gently bring to the boil. Lower the heat and simmer for 10 minutes. Set aside to cool a little, then strain, discarding the spices and bay leaf.

3 Open each herring and spread it with mustard. Set 1 tablespoon of the shallots aside, and arrange the remainder in a line down the middle of each fish. Roll up from head to tail and secure with a cocktail stick.

4 Put the herrings in an ovenproof dish and pour over the strained marinade. Sprinkle with the reserved shallots, cover and bake for 15 minutes. Allow to cool. Leave to souse in the fridge for at least 2 days. Serve with rye bread.

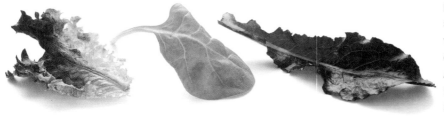

dinner recipes

roast tomato and red pepper soup

serves 4

8 ripe medium tomatoes, cut in half
4 large red peppers, cut in half and
    deseeded
4 garlic cloves
½ tbsp olive oil, plus extra for drizzling
1 onion, chopped
600ml/1pt/2½ cups vegetable stock (see
    page 109) or water
Freshly squeezed juice of 1 lemon
Freshly ground black pepper
1 handful fresh flat-leaf parsley, roughly
    chopped, to serve

1 Preheat the oven to
   190°C/375°F/Gas 5.
2 Put the tomatoes cut-side up
   on a baking sheet, together
   with the red pepper and garlic.
   Drizzle with oil and bake for 30
   minutes.
3 Heat ½ tablespoon oil in a pan,
   add the onion and cook until
   soft. Add the tomatoes, red
   peppers, garlic and stock. Bring
   to the boil, then simmer for 15
   minutes. Allow to cool a little,
   then purée in a blender.
4 Return to the pan and heat
   through. Stir in the lemon juice,
   season with black pepper and
   serve sprinkled with parsley.

french onion soup

serves 4

2 tbsp olive oil
4 large onions, thinly sliced
2 garlic cloves, crushed
1l/35fl oz/4 cups vegetable stock (see
    page 109) or water
1 sprig rosemary
1 sprig thyme
1 bay leaf
Freshly ground black pepper
1 handful fresh flat-leaf parsley, roughly
    chopped, to serve

1 Heat the oil in a large saucepan. Add the onions
   and garlic and cook over
   medium-high heat until they
   start to colour.
2 Pour in the stock, rosemary,
   thyme and bay leaf. Bring to
   the boil, lower the heat and
   leave to simmer for 30 minutes. Remove the herbs,
   season to taste with black
   pepper and serve sprinkled
   with parsley.

sea bass with lime and coriander

serves 4

4 sea bass fillets, about 200g/7oz each
Freshly squeezed juice of 2 limes
2 tbsp olive oil
2 garlic cloves, crushed
1 handful fresh coriander leaves,
    roughly chopped
1 lime, sliced, to serve

1 Put the sea bass fillets in a
   single layer in a shallow, heat-
   proof dish. Mix together the
   lime juice, oil, garlic and coriander leaves and pour over the
   fish. Leave to marinate in the
   fridge for at least 30 minutes.
   Meanwhile, preheat the grill to
   medium-hot.
2 Grill the fish in the dish for 10
   minutes until the flesh is just
   firm. Baste the fish frequently
   with the lime and coriander
   marinade while grilling. Serve
   with the lime slices on the side.

cinnamon aubergines

. . . .

serves 4

2 large aubergines
2 tbsp olive oil
2 large onions
4 cloves garlic
2 large tomatoes, skinned, deseeded
  and chopped
½ tsp acacia honey
12 fresh basil leaves, torn
½ tsp ground cinnamon
Grated zest and freshly squeezed juice
  of 1 unwaxed lemon
1 handful chopped almonds
Freshly ground black pepper

1 Preheat the oven to
   180°C/350°F/Gas 4.
2 Put the aubergines in a large
   pan and cover with boiling
   water. Return to the boil and
   cook for 10 minutes. Drain,
   then plunge into cold water
   to cool. Cut each aubergine
   in half lengthways. Scoop out
   and reserve most of the flesh,
   leaving a 1cm/½in thick shell.
   Lightly oil the insides of the
   aubergine shells and season
   with black pepper. Put on a
   greased baking sheet and bake
   for 30 minutes.
3 Meanwhile, chop the aubergine
   flesh and set aside. Heat the
   remaining oil in a frying pan,
   add the onion and garlic and
   cook for about 5 minutes, until
   soft. Add the tomatoes, honey,

basil and cinnamon and leave
to simmer for 15 minutes. Add
the aubergine flesh, lemon
juice and zest, and almonds and
cook for a further 10 minutes.
Season with black pepper.
4 Remove the aubergine shells
   from the oven, and fill with the
   hot tomato and aubergine
   mixture. Serve half an aubergine to each person.

stuffed vine leaves with tzatziki

. . . .

serves 4

20 vine leaves, fresh or tinned
½ tbsp olive oil
3 shallots, finely chopped
4 garlic cloves, crushed
125g/4½oz/scant ⅔ cup brown rice,
  rinsed and drained
3 tbsp sultanas
3 tbsp flaked almonds
Grated zest and freshly squeezed juice
  of 1 unwaxed lemon
850ml/1½pt/3½ cups vegetable stock
  (see page 109) or water
6 spring onions, finely chopped
1 handful fresh mint leaves, roughly
  chopped
1 handful fresh flat-leaf parsley, roughly
  chopped
Freshly ground black pepper

For the tzatziki:
1 cucumber, peeled and coarsely grated
200ml/7fl oz/¾ cup low-fat bio yogurt
2 garlic cloves, crushed
1 handful fresh mint leaves finely chopped

Grated zest and freshly squeezed juice
  of 1 unwaxed lemon

1 If using fresh vine leaves,
   plunge them into boiling water
   for 1 minute. Drain and remove
   the coarse stalks. If using
   tinned leaves, rinse them under
   cold running water.
2 Heat the oil in a large pan.
   Add the shallots and garlic and
   cook for about 5 minutes. Add
   the rice, sultanas, almonds
   and lemon zest and cook for 1
   minute. Add enough stock to
   cover the rice. Cook until the
   rice is tender. Leave to cool,
   then stir in the spring onions,
   mint and parsley. Season with
   pepper.
3 Put a spoonful of the rice mixture on each vine leaf and fold
   the leaf around it to make a
   parcel. Pack the parcels tightly
   in a pan. Cover with stock and
   sprinkle with the lemon juice.
   Put a plate on top of the parcels to keep them submerged.
   Cover with a lid or foil, and
   simmer over very gentle heat
   for 50 minutes.
4 Make the tzatziki by mixing all
   the ingredients. Season with
   black pepper. Serve the stuffed
   vine leaves with the tzatziki
   as a dip.

right: cinnamon aubergines

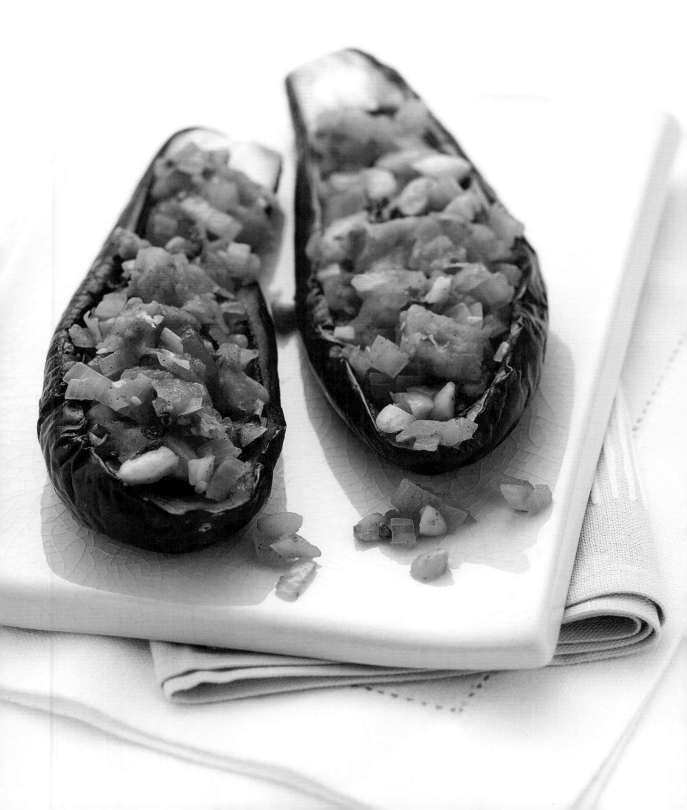

roasted red peppers with herby bulgur wheat

serves 4

2 large red peppers, cut in half lengthways, cored and deseeded (stalks
   intact)
2 large orange peppers, cut in half
   lengthways, cored and deseeded
   (stalks intact)
2 tbsp olive oil
16 cherry tomatoes, cut in half
125ml/4fl oz/½ cup low-fat fromage frais
4 tbsp pesto
2 garlic cloves, crushed
2 tbsp pine nuts
Freshly ground black pepper

For the herby bulgur wheat:
125g/4½oz/1 cup bulgur wheat
750ml/26fl oz/3 cups vegetable stock
   (see page 109) or water
Grated zest and freshly squeezed juice
   of 1 unwaxed lemon
1 small handful fresh coriander leaves,
   finely chopped
1 small handful fresh mint leaves, finely
   chopped
1 small handful fresh flat-leaf parsley,
   finely chopped
12 fresh basil leaves, torn
4 spring onions, finely chopped

1 Preheat the oven to
   180°C/350°F/Gas 4.
2 Put the peppers cut-side up on
   a baking sheet and lightly brush
   with oil. Put 4 tomato halves in
   each pepper half.
3 Mash together the fromage
   frais, pesto and garlic and

spoon over the tomatoes in
each pepper half. Season to
taste with black pepper and
sprinkle over the pine nuts.
Drizzle with a little more oil
and roast in the oven for 45
minutes, until the pepper skins
start to char.

4 Meanwhile, put the bulgur
   wheat and stock in a large pan
   and bring to the boil. Lower
   the heat and simmer gently for
   about 10 minutes, until all the
   liquid is absorbed. Stir in the
   lemon juice and zest, herbs and
   spring onions. Serve one red
   and one orange pepper half
   per person with a side helping
   of herby bulgur wheat.

stir-fried turkey with bean sprouts

serves 4

For the marinade:
2 tbsp low-sodium soy sauce
3 tsp dry sherry
3 tsp olive oil
3 tsp clear honey
Freshly squeezed juice of 1 orange
2 garlic cloves, crushed
5cm/2in piece fresh ginger, peeled and
   grated

4 skinless turkey breast fillets, about
   200g/7oz each
3 tbsp olive oil or unrefined virgin
   coconut oil

4 spring onions, chopped
1 handful bean sprouts
125g/4½oz white cabbage, shredded
1 handful green beans, trimmed
1 tbsp toasted sesame seeds
Freshly ground black pepper

1 Put all the marinade ingredients
   in a screw-top jar and shake
   vigorously to mix well. Lay the
   turkey fillets in a shallow heat-
   proof dish and pour over half
   the marinade. Turn the fillets
   to coat them and leave to marinate for at least 30 minutes.
   Preheat the grill to medium-hot.
2 Grill the turkey in the dish for
   10–15 minutes. Turn the fillets
   halfway through cooking. Heat
   the oil in a large frying pan.
   Add the spring onions, bean
   sprouts, cabbage and green
   beans and stir-fry for 3 minutes.
   Pour in the remaining marinade
   and stir-fry for 2 minutes.
3 Divide the stir-fry between four
   serving plates. Place a grilled
   turkey fillet on top of each
   portion and sprinkle over the
   sesame seeds. Season with
   black pepper and serve.

mushroom and walnut lasagne

serves 4

1 tbsp olive oil
250g/9oz onions, chopped
250g/9oz carrots, chopped
4 garlic cloves
6 celery stalks, chopped
1 handful mixed fresh herbs, such as
    thyme, parsley, oregano and rose-
    mary, roughly chopped
3 ripe medium tomatoes, skinned,
    deseeded and chopped, plus 1
    medium tomato, thinly sliced
300g/10½oz mushrooms, sliced
1 handful walnut pieces
Freshly ground black pepper
12 sheets easy-cook spinach or
    wholemeal lasagne sheets
250ml/9fl oz/1 cup low-fat fromage frais
200g/7oz mozzarella cheese, grated

1 Preheat the oven to
   180°C/350°F/Gas 4.
2 Heat the oil in a large frying
   pan. Add the onions, carrots,
   garlic, celery and chopped
   herbs and cook over medium
   heat for 10 minutes. Stir in the
   chopped tomatoes, mushrooms and walnut pieces and
   cook for a further 10 minutes.
   Season with black pepper.
3 Spread one third of the mushroom and walnut mixture over
   the base of an oven-proof
   dish. Cover with three lasagne sheets, then spread these
   with one third of the fromage
   frais. Repeat these layers twice
   more. Top with the cheese and
   sliced tomato. Bake for 45
   minutes and serve.

rosé trout

serves 4

4 trout fillets, about 175g/6oz each
2 shallots, sliced into rings
375ml/13fl oz/1½ cups rosé wine
1 handful flaked almonds
Freshly ground black pepper
1 handful fresh dill, roughly chopped,
    to serve

1 Preheat the oven to
   180°C/350°F/Gas 4.
2 Put the trout fillets in a single
   layer in an oven-proof dish.
   Sprinkle the shallots over the
   top and pour over the wine.
   Scatter over the almonds, cover
   and bake for about 30 minutes,
   until the fillets are cooked.
   Serve immediately, sprinkled
   with the dill.

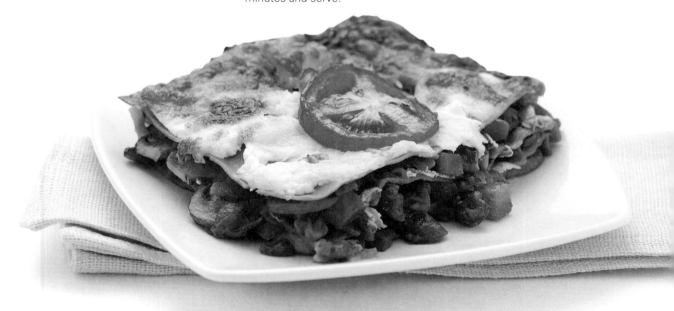

mushroom and walnut lasagne

grilled mushrooms with almonds and basil

. . . .

serves 4

4 tbsp olive oil
2 garlic cloves
2 spring onions, chopped
1 handful flaked almonds
1 handful mixed seeds, such as
    pumpkin, sunflower and sesame
4 large flat mushrooms
1 handful wholemeal breadcrumbs
1 handful fresh basil leaves, roughly
    chopped
Freshly ground black pepper

1 Preheat the oven to
    180°C/350°F/Gas 4.
2 Heat the oil in a frying pan. Add
    the garlic and spring onions
    and cook over medium heat for
    about 4 minutes until soft. Add
    the flaked almonds and mixed
    seeds and cook for a further
    minute, stirring.
3 Put the mushrooms hollow-side
    up in a shallow oven-proof dish.
    Spoon the almond and seed
    mixture into the mushrooms.
    Sprinkle over the breadcrumbs
    and basil and season with black
    pepper. Cover with foil and
    bake for 15 minutes. Serve
    immediately.

dessert recipes

oatmeal flummery

. . . .

serves 4

2 handfuls porridge oats
1 handful blanched almonds, roughly
    chopped
1 handful walnuts, roughly chopped
250g/9oz silken tofu
2 ripe bananas, peeled and sliced
Grated zest and freshly squeezed juice
    of 1 unwaxed lemon
1 tbsp clear honey (optional)

1 Lightly toast the oats and nuts
    under the grill. Leave to cool.
2 Mash together the other
    ingredients, then chill them.
    Fold in the oats/nuts and serve.

mulled fruit salad

. . . .

serves 4

4 ripe peaches, cut in half, stoned and
    sliced
8 fresh apricots, cut in half and stoned
    (or 8 dried, ready-to-eat apricots)
150ml/5fl oz/½ cup freshly squeezed
    orange juice
150ml/5fl oz/1⅓ glasses light red wine,
    such as Beaujolais
½ tsp cinnamon powder
1 handful raisins
2 bananas, peeled and thickly sliced

1 Simmer all the ingredients in a
    pan for 10 minutes.
2 Serve warm.

creamy turkish delight figs

. . . .

serves 4

250g/9oz silken tofu
Grated zest and freshly squeezed juice
    of 1 unwaxed orange
3 tsp clear honey
12 ripe fresh figs
1–2 tbsp rosewater, for drizzling

1 Blend the tofu, orange juice
    and honey in a blender.
2 Cut a cross in the top of each
    fig. Spoon the tofu into the
    figs. Sprinkle with orange zest
    and drizzle with rosewater.

walnut and fruit compote

. . . .

serves 4

1 small, ripe Galia melon, deseeded and
    flesh divided into balls
1 red grapefruit, divided into segments
1 large banana, peeled and sliced
150ml/5fl oz/⅔ cup unsweetened apple
    juice
1 handful walnuts, roughly chopped

1 Halve each grapefruit segment
    lengthways. Remove and dis-
    card the outer membranes.
2 Put all the fruit in a bowl. Add
    the apple juice and walnuts
    and serve.

bites, snacks and drinks

toasted mixed nuts

serves 4

1 handful blanched almonds
1 handful hazelnuts
1 handful unsalted cashew nuts
1 handful walnuts
1 handful Brazil nuts
1 handful raisins (optional)

1 Warm a large frying pan over medium heat. Toast the nuts gently, moving and shaking the pan as they turn golden. Take care not to burn them.
2 Let the nuts cool. Mix with the raisins, if using, and serve.

chickpea and avocado hummus

serves 4

400g/14oz tin chickpeas, drained
1 large ripe avocado
2 garlic cloves, crushed
Freshly squeezed juice of 1 lemon
Freshly ground black pepper
1 handful fresh mint leaves
Oatcakes or rice cakes, to serve

1 Put all the ingredients in a blender (except the oatcakes) and process until smooth.
2 Serve with oatcakes.

mock caviar

serves 4

2 medium aubergines, cut in half lengthways
2 spring onions, finely chopped
2 garlic cloves, crushed
Freshly squeezed juice of 1 lemon
12 fresh basil leaves
4 tbsp extra virgin olive oil
Freshly ground black pepper

1 Preheat the oven to 200°C/400°F/Gas 6.
2 Put the aubergines cut-side down on a baking sheet. Bake for 30 minutes. Allow to cool slightly, then scoop out the pulp into a bowl and discard the skin.
3 Place the aubergine pulp in a blender with the spring onions, garlic, lemon juice, basil leaves and oil. Process until smooth and well blended. Season with black pepper and serve.

berry smoothie

serves 4

4 handfuls mixed berries, such as blackberries, raspberries, strawberries and blueberries
600ml/1pt/2½ cups low-fat bio yogurt or fromage frais
1 tbsp mixed seeds, such as pumpkin, sunflower and sesame
2 tbsp crushed ice
A little honey (optional)

1 Blend all the ingredients in a blender until smooth. If you wish, you can sweeten with a little honey.
2 Pour into tall glasses and serve.

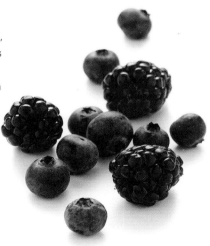

introducing the full-strength program

The full-strength program is designed to bring your blood pressure down as efficiently as possible. It's ideal for people who have completed the moderate program and wish to move on to a more advanced program; and for those who want to obtain the maximum beneficial effects for their hypertension and the health of their cardiovascular system. You need to be fit and healthy, and already eat a well-balanced diet with plenty of fresh fruit and vegetables.

There are 14 daily plans that you can repeat to create a 28-day program. Follow the full-strength program for at least a month before assessing its benefits. Once you feel comfortable with the diet and lifestyle changes involved, feel free to make your own adjustments that take into account your personal likes, dislikes and lifestyle.

The full-strength program diet

The diet incorporates foods identified in the *British Medical Journal* as having the most beneficial influence on the risk of heart attack and stroke, and which have the potential to increase life expectancy by six and a half years for men, and almost five years for women if eaten on a regular basis. The diet includes a high intake of almonds, garlic, dark chocolate, fruit and vegetables, plus fish three to four times a week. These superfoods were selected on the basis of evidence pooled from a number of scientific trials. Each of the key ingredients stands up on its own merit rather than as part of a particular type of diet, such as the Mediterranean diet. Although the foods are similar to those found in the

gentle and moderate programs, they are consumed with higher frequency.

If you are hypertensive but not on anti-hypertensive medication, you can expect to reduce your blood pressure by at least 9/4mmHg on the full-strength program. And if you also take the recommended supplements, you may be able to lower your blood pressure by 15/8 mmHg or more over the course of one month. If you are taking anti-hypertensive drugs, the full-strength diet and supplement program will improve their effectiveness. It will also lower your total and LDL-cholesterol levels and reduce your triglyceride levels (see page 51).

As I recommended in the gentle and moderate programs, dispose of any foods in your cupboards that are high in sugar, salt, saturated fat and trans fats. Do not add salt (sodium chloride) during cooking or at the table. Obtain flavour from fresh herbs and black pepper instead. If you haven't yet started to make your own fruit and vegetable juices at home (see pages 111–112), now is the time to start.

Including chocolate and wine in your diet Although you may feel that eating chocolate and drinking red wine runs counter to conventional wisdom, the evidence for their positive effect on hypertension is strong. Dark chocolate (at least 70 percent cocoa solids) contains powerful antioxidant polyphenols that are similar to those found in red wine and green tea.

Of all the superfoods, red wine has the most blood pressure-lowering benefits – but only when drunk in moderation. More than 150ml (5fl oz) a day can have a

Shopping list

You will need all the food and drink items on the shopping list for the gentle program (see page 80). In addition, you will need the following (where possible, buy regularly in small quantities for optimum freshness).

dairy and soy products
buffalo mozzarella cheese
firm tofu
silken tofu

fruit and vegetables
blueberries
butternut squash or pumpkin
cooking apples
dried cranberries
guava
raspberries
strawberries

herbs and spices
dill
fennel seeds
green peppercorns
lemongrass

grains
barley bread
coarse oatmeal
hemp or spinach tagliatelle, lasagne or spaghetti
red rice
soy bread
wild rice

proteins
butter beans
chickpeas
green lentils
herrings
lean pork fillets
sea bass

miscellaneous
coconut milk

harmful effect on health. Scientists have found that the highest content of beneficial antioxidants is found in wine made from Cabernet Sauvignon grapes. And, compared with red wines from other parts of the world, researchers from Glasgow University found that Cabernet Sauvignons from Chile have the highest amount of heart-friendly anti-oxidant flavonols. Narrowing things down even further, they found that Cabernet Sauvignons from the Viña MontGras estate have significantly more antioxidants than any other Chilean wine tested.

The full-strength program exercise routine

The full-strength exercise program is designed for those who are relatively fit and who already exercise regularly for 45 minutes on most days. During the program, I recommend that you increase the level of exercise you take to 45–60 minutes a day on at least five days a week. Try to find new forms of exercise so you build variety into your exercise program – that way you won't get bored. Perform stretch and weight exercises on the other two days so you are exercising most days or every day. As well as brisk walking, cycling and swimming, consider bowling, golf and similar activities that improve your social life as well as your health. Here are some other ways to be active:

- Walk rather than drive your children to school and then gently jog home.
- Whenever you walk anywhere – indoors as well as outdoors – do so at a brisk pace.
- When you are doing manual chores (such as DIY or housework), do them as vigorously as possible.
- Reduce time spent on sedentary activities such as watching television and instead go for a bike ride or walk with friends, family or even a borrowed dog if you don't own one yourself.

Full-strength program supplements

These are the supplements I recommend you take while you are following the full-strength program. You can buy them from pharmacies, supermarkets and healthfood stores. Read about these supplements and how they lower your blood pressure on pages 60–63.

recommended daily supplements

- Vitamin C (2000mg)
- Vitamin E (800i.u/536mg)
- Lycopene carotenoid complex (15mg)
- Selenium (200mcg)
- Co-enzyme Q10 (120mg)
- Garlic tablets (allicin yield 1000–1500mcg)
- Omega-3 fish oil (900mg daily; for example, 3x1g fish oil capsules, each supplying 180mg EPA plus 120mg DHA)

optional daily supplements (these will provide additional health benefits)

- Alpha lipoic acid (300mg). May be combined with L-carnitine in a 1:1 ratio
- Magnesium (300mg)
- Calcium (1000mg)
- Folic acid (1000mcg) plus vitamin B12 (50mcg)
- Reishi (1500mg)
- Bilberry fruit extracts (180mg; standardized to give 25 percent anthocyanins)
- Probiotics (fermented milk drinks, bio yogurt or supplements)

- Use the stairs rather than the lift or escalator.
- Walk part or all of the way to your destinations – get off the bus/train one stop earlier than normal.

If you miss a day's exercise due to illness or time constraints, don't feel you've failed (exercise routines are at risk of lapsing after an unexpected interruption). Rather than giving up, resolve to get back to exercising as quickly as possible – plan exactly what you're going to do and when and don't let your slot of exercise time get filled up with a different activity – even if the other activity seems more pressing.

Whenever you are exercising, always warm up and cool down and, if you are cycling outdoors, wear appropriate safety equipment. Always monitor your 10-second pulse rate (see page 69) to ensure you are not overdoing it. The exercise routines in the full-strength program are more intense than in the previous two

programs, so if you are in any doubt about your fitness, or if you have angina or a history of heart attack, ask your doctor for guidance on how much exercise you can take. Stop exercising at once if you feel unwell.

The full-strength program therapies

The full-strength program includes relaxation techniques such as transcendental meditation and practitioner-led therapies such as naturopathy and acupuncture. If you are new to meditation, you may find that it's difficult to focus your mind at first. Whether you sit in quiet contemplation or focus on a mantra or a yantra, your mind may be full of busy chatter. This is normal. In time, however, you will find that the discipline of meditation helps mental chatter to lessen.

You will need to book two appointments with complementary therapists in advance – please look at days seven and fourteen of the program now.

1

the full-strength program day one

Daily menu

- **Breakfast: stuffed tomatoes (see page 165)**

- **Morning snack: a portion of super-food fruit (see pages 56–59), such as apple, blueberries, cherries, figs, grapes, kiwi, guava, mango or pomegranate**

- **Lunch: almond trout (see page 167). Bowl of mixed salad leaves sprinkled with walnuts, pumpkin seeds, chopped garlic, walnut oil and red wine vinegar. Fresh fruit**

- **Afternoon snack: a handful of almonds**

- **Dinner: grilled salmon steak marinated in olive oil and lime juice. Broccoli. Brown rice. 40–50g (about 1½oz) bar dark chocolate**

- **Drinks: 570ml (1pt) semi-skimmed or skimmed milk. Freshly squeezed fruit/veg juice. Unlimited green/black or white tea, herbal tea and mineral water. 150ml (5fl oz) red wine or unsweetened red grape juice**

- **Supplements: see page 145**

Over the next 14 days, I introduce you to a series of yoga postures that form a sequence known as the sun salutation. Regular yoga practice can lower systolic blood pressure by 10–15mmHg.

Daily exercise routine

When you get up in the morning do the first posture of the sun salutation (see below). Walk briskly for 30–45 minutes during the day. Alternatively, swim or cycle for 20 minutes. In the evening, unwind by lying in the corpse pose (see page 97) for 15 minutes.

Sun salutation – 1st posture

1 Stand tall and straight with your feet together. Bend your elbows and bring your palms together in front of your chest in a prayer-like position.

2 Relax in this position for one minute. As you breathe in and out, visualize the sun rising. Imagine its warmth and light radiating through your body.

Meditation

Daily meditation can lower average systolic blood pressure by at least 10mmHg within 12 weeks. During

the first week, I suggest you meditate once a day for 10–20 minutes, always before a meal, such as breakfast or dinner. Then build up to meditating twice a day.

Going-inward meditation

1 Start your first meditation session by sitting in a comfortable position near a non-ticking clock or watch. Close your eyes. Breathe slowly and naturally and allow your mind to empty.

2 Over the next 10 minutes, direct your consciousness inward, deeper and deeper, to a place of utter calm and peace.

3 Open your eyes. Remain seated for at least a minute.

Avoid inversion

The yoga sequence in this program includes some head-down poses that are not recommended if your blood pressure is 160/100mmHg or higher. If this applies to you, follow the gentle or moderate program until your blood pressure is lower.

day two

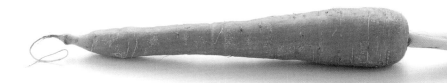

Daily menu

- **Breakfast: home-made muesli (see page 100) topped with banana and coconut shavings**

- **Morning snack: a portion of super-food fruit (see day one)**

- **Lunch: beetroot and tofu medley (see page 166). Bowl of mixed salad leaves sprinkled with grated carrot, Brazil nuts, pumpkin seeds and Mediterranean herb oil (see page 168)**

- **Afternoon snack: a handful of almonds**

- **Dinner: winter vegetable stew with rosemary (see page 170). Almond chocolate cups (see page 172)**

- **Drinks: 570ml (1pt) semi-skimmed or skimmed milk. Freshly squeezed fruit/veg juice. Unlimited green/black or white tea, herbal tea and mineral water. 150ml (5fl oz) red wine or unsweetened red grape juice**

- **Supplements: see page 145**

Daily exercise routine

When you get up in the morning do the first posture of the sun salutation (see day one) followed by the next posture (see below). Walk briskly for 30–45 minutes during the day. Alternatively, swim or cycle for 20 minutes. In the evening, unwind by lying in the corpse pose (see page 97).

Sun salutation – 2nd posture

1 As you inhale, raise your arms out to the sides and then up in a wide circle. Let your palms meet over your head and your fingers point up.
2 Let your chest open and expand as your arms lift. Press your palms firmly together and look up at them.
3 Keeping your feet flat on the floor, stretch your arms up above your head so you are as tall as possible. Slowly bend back as far as is comfortable. Hold your breath and stay in this position for a few seconds, letting your mind empty.

Meditation

As well as performing the basic meditation that you did yesterday,

I'd now like you to focus on your breathing – this will enable you to get into a meditative state more quickly.

Breath meditation

1 Sit quietly and comfortably with your eyes closed. Breathe in slowly and deeply through your nose, and then out through your mouth.
2 Focus your attention on how cool the air feels when you inhale, and how warm it feels when you breathe out.
3 With each out-breath, imagine tension leaving your body. Feel yourself become more and more relaxed with each breath.
4 Start counting your breaths, saying the number of each breath as you let it go. This gives you something to focus on and helps to stop thoughts distracting you.
5 Now switch to breathing in through your mouth, and out through your nose. Decide which pattern of breathing feels most comfortable for you and continue this for the rest of today's meditation. Meditate for 10–20 minutes.

the full-strength program day three

Daily menu

- Breakfast: herrings in oatmeal (see page 164). Grilled tomato. Wholemeal or rye toast

- Morning snack: a portion of superfood fruit (see day one)

- Lunch: bowl of mixed salad leaves sprinkled with sprouted beans, beetroot, carrot, red pepper, walnuts, pumpkin seeds, chopped garlic, walnut oil and red wine vinegar. Wholemeal roll. Low-fat bio yogurt with fresh fruit

- Afternoon snack: a handful of almonds

- Dinner: Mediterranean mackerel (see page 171). Wholemeal or hemp pasta. Broccoli. Baked apples (see page 173) with low-fat fromage frais

- Drinks: 570ml (1pt) semi-skimmed or skimmed milk. Freshly squeezed fruit/veg juice. Unlimited green/black or white tea, herbal tea and mineral water. 150ml (5fl oz) red wine or unsweetened red grape juice

- Supplements: see page 145

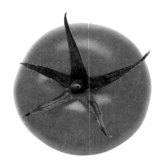

Daily exercise routine

When you get up in the morning do the first two postures of the sun salutation (see days one and two) followed by the posture below. Walk briskly for 30–45 minutes during the day. Alternatively, swim or cycle for 20 minutes. In the evening, unwind by lying in the corpse pose (see page 97) for 15 minutes.

Sun salutation – 3rd posture

1 Breathe out and bend forward from your waist, keeping your arms straight out in front of you, and your palms together.

2 Bend as low as you can while keeping your back straight. Tuck your head in. Hold this position as long as feels comfortable, breathing in and out gently through your nose.

Meditation

Today, I'd like you to practise either of the meditations you have learned in the previous two days. But, beforehand, I'd like you to practise a yogic breathing exercise called sitkari (folded-up tongue). This technique "cools" the mind and helps you get into a meditative state more quickly.

Sitkari pranayama

1 Sit quietly and comfortably, with your back straight and your eyes closed. Start by breathing in, slowly and deeply, through your mouth, then out through both nostrils.

2 Fold your tongue back and press the tip of your tongue against the roof of your mouth. This leaves a narrow opening on either side of your tongue.

3 Inhale through these side openings – make a hissing sound with your breath. Continue to breathe out, slowly and deeply, through your nose. Repeat this several times.

4 When you are ready, return to normal, slow rhythmic breathing. Let your mind empty for your chosen meditation.

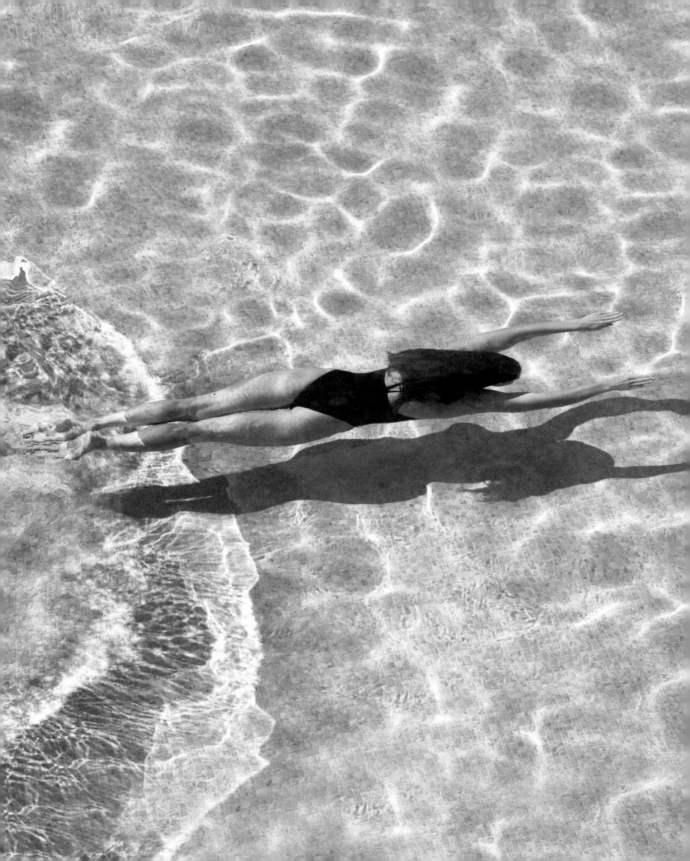

the full-strength program day four

Daily menu

- **Breakfast: porridge with Brazil nuts and apricots**
- **Morning snack: a portion of superfood fruit (see day one)**
- **Lunch: almond and broccoli salad (see page 166) served with mixed salad leaves sprinkled with pumpkin seeds and Mediterranean herb oil (see page 168). Wholemeal roll. Low-fat bio yogurt with fresh fruit**
- **Afternoon snack: chocolate florentines (see page 173)**
- **Dinner: lemon pork (see page 171). Spinach. Wholemeal or hemp pasta. 40–50g (about 1½oz) bar dark chocolate**
- **Drinks: 570ml (1pt) semi-skimmed or skimmed milk. Freshly squeezed fruit/veg juice. Unlimited green/black or white tea, herbal tea and mineral water. 150ml (5fl oz) red wine or unsweetened red grape juice**
- **Supplements: see page 145**

Today you are going to meditate on a yantra, an ancient geometric design that, because of its shape, is believed to act as a doorway to higher universal energies and bring you closer to enlightenment. Yantra designs are many thousands of years old. Unlike other geometric designs that are used in meditation, such as mandalas, yantras are revealed to the world by a clairvoyant tantric guru – you cannot make one up. The chatter of the mind quickly ceases when you focus on a yantra during meditation.

Daily exercise routine

When you get up in the morning do the first three postures of the sun salutation (see days one to three) followed by the posture below. Walk briskly for 30–45 minutes or swim or cycle for 20 minutes during the day. In the evening, unwind in corpse pose (see page 97) for 15 minutes.

Sun salutation – 4th posture

1 From the third posture fold forward further to grasp the backs of your ankles or calves (or as far down your leg as you can)
2 Tuck your chin in and bend your elbows to pull your upper body gently in toward your legs.
3 Breathe out and hold your breath for a few seconds.

Meditation

Select a yantra to which you feel drawn (images and posters are available on the internet). Place the image so that its centre is at eye level when you sit down.

Yantra meditation

1 Focus on the centre of the yantra. Now widen your area of focus so you can see the whole design.
2 When you feel ready, close your eyes and picture the yantra in your mind. Repeat these steps for 10–15 minutes.

Meditation postures

Good postures for meditation include sitting upright in a straight-backed chair or sitting cross-legged on the floor with your hands resting in your lap or on your knees.

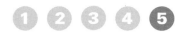

day five

Daily menu

- **Breakfast: grilled tomatoes sprinkled with thyme. Wholegrain, rye, soy or barley toast**

- **Morning snack: a portion of superfood fruit (see day one)**

- **Lunch: green minestrone (see page 166). Wholemeal roll. Low-fat bio yogurt with fresh fruit**

- **Afternoon snack: a handful of almonds**

- **Dinner: mackerel and cucumber in wine (see page 171). Brown rice mixed with wild rice. Chocolate petit fours (see page 173)**

- **Drinks: 570ml (1pt) semi-skimmed or skimmed milk. Freshly squeezed fruit/veg juice. Unlimited green/black or white tea, herbal tea and mineral water. 150ml (5fl oz) red wine or unsweetened red grape juice**

- **Supplements: see page 145**

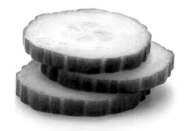

Today's dinner provides an excellent source of omega-3 fatty acids, selenium and vitamins B3, B6 and B12 in the form of mackerel. Weight for weight, mackerel provides more omega-3 fatty acids than any other oily fish. Research shows that eating mackerel three times a week over an eight-month period significantly lowered both systolic and diastolic blood pressure in a group of people with essential hypertension.

Daily exercise routine

When you get up, do the first four postures of the sun salutation (see days one to four) followed by the posture below. Walk briskly for 30–45 minutes during the day. Alternatively, swim or cycle for 20 minutes. In the evening, unwind by lying in the corpse pose (see page 97) for 15 minutes.

Sun salutation – 5th posture

1 Following on from the fourth posture, breathe in, let go of your legs and stand up straight.
2 As you breathe out, step forward as far as you can with your right leg, bend your right knee and place both hands on the floor, arms straight, on either side of your right foot. As you come forward onto the ball of your left foot, keep your left knee off the floor.
3 Tilt your head back to look up. The next time you do this exercise, lunge forward with your left foot instead.

Meditation

Today I'd like you to select a personal mantra – a word or phrase to say to yourself as you breathe out. A mantra helps you reach a higher state of consciousness.

Mantra meditation

1 Choose a word that reflects your spiritual beliefs (for example, "Amen" or "Shalom"), a sound that you are instinctively drawn to (for example, "om" or "aaaaaaah"), or a word or phrase that you find helpful (for example, "let go" or "calm").
2 Close your eyes and sit quietly, gently breathing in through your nose, and out through your mouth. Start whispering your mantra on each out-breath in a soft, rhythmic and relaxed way. Do this for 10–15 minutes.

the full-strength program day six

Daily menu

- **Breakfast: blueberry and almond mousse (see page 164). Slice of wholemeal, rye, soy or barley toast**

- **Morning snack: a portion of superfood fruit (see day one)**

- **Lunch: cheese, fruit and nut platter (see page 167). Bowl of mixed salad leaves sprinkled with Brazil nuts, pumpkin seeds, chopped garlic, walnut oil and red wine vinegar. Low-fat bio yogurt**

- **Afternoon snack: a handful of almonds**

- **Dinner: chickpea curry (see page 170). Almond rice (see page 170). 40–50g (about 1½oz) bar dark chocolate**

- **Drinks: 570ml (1pt) semi-skimmed or skimmed milk. Freshly squeezed fruit/veg juice. Unlimited green/black or white tea, herbal tea and mineral water. 150ml (5fl oz) red wine or unsweetened red grape juice**

- **Supplements: see page 145**

Daily exercise routine

When you get up in the morning do the first five postures of the sun salutation (see days one to five) followed by the posture below. Walk briskly for 30–45 minutes or swim or cycle for 20 minutes during the day. In the evening, unwind by lying in the corpse pose (see page 97) for 15 minutes.

Sun salutation – 6th posture

1 From the fifth posture, straighten your upper body and gently move your arms out to the side and up.
2 Bring your palms together over your head, fingers pointing to the sky. Look up at your hands.
3 Hold your breath in this position for a few seconds. Keep your mind as empty as possible.

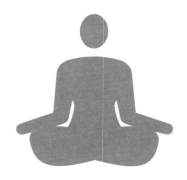

Meditation

Today you are going to meditate on the chakras – seven energy centres within your subtle body (see page 43).

Chakra meditation

1 Start by meditating on the first chakra, the root chakra, by bringing your awareness to the base of your spine and visualizing the colour red.
2 Move your awareness to your sacral chaka (at your sacrum) and imagine the colour orange.
3 Move up to the next chakra, the solar plexus. Imagine a yellow colour here.
4 Focus on the centre of your chest – your heart chakra – and visualize the colour green.
5 Move your awareness to your throat. Imagine sky blue.
6 Focus on the sixth chakra between your eyes, the brow chakra. Visualize indigo.
7 Finally, visualize the colour violet at the top of your head (your crown chakra). Then imagine white light expanding from this chakra and enveloping you in a sphere of energy. Enjoy the feeling of calm and peace.

day seven

Daily menu

- **Breakfast: Windward Islands trout (see page 164). Slice of whole-meal, rye, soy or barley toast**

- **Morning snack: a portion of superfood fruit (see day one)**

- **Lunch: bowl of mixed salad leaves sprinkled with grated carrot, beetroot, bean sprouts, sliced button mushrooms and Mediterranean herb oil (see page 168). Wholemeal roll. Low-fat yogurt with fresh fruit**

- **Afternoon snack: toasted almonds with seeds (see page 173)**

- **Dinner: oriental tofu stir-fry (see page 168). Red rice. A piece of fresh fruit**

- **Drinks: 570ml (1pt) semi-skimmed or skimmed milk. Freshly squeezed fruit/veg juice. Unlimited green/black or white tea, herbal tea and mineral water. 150ml (5fl oz) red wine or unsweetened red grape juice**

- **Supplements: see page 145**

Daily exercise routine

When you get up in the morning do the first six postures of the sun salutation (see days one to six) followed by the posture below. Walk briskly for 30–45 minutes or swim or cycle for 20 minutes. In the evening, unwind by lying in the corpse pose (see page 97) for 15 minutes.

Sun salutation – 7th posture

1 Following straight on from the last posture, breathe out and bring both hands down onto the floor on either side of your right foot.

2 Step back with your right foot so that both feet are together. Straighten your body so that you are in the straight-backed plank position (see page 121).

Slow breathing

If you feel stressed, make a conscious effort to slow down your breathing. Imagine a candle in front of your face. Exhale slowly – so that the candle just flickers slightly.

3 Hold this position for as long as is comfortable, breathing gently in and out, keeping your mind as quiet as possible.

Consulting a naturopath

Now you are halfway through the program, I suggest you see a naturopath. To find an accredited naturopath, see page 175. Many are trained in homeopathy, herbal medicine, chiropractic and osteopathy as well as nutritional medicine. During the first consultation, a naturopath will ask questions about your past and current health, and perform a medical examination that includes checking your blood pressure, listening to your heart and lungs and, sometimes, examining your irises. He or she may also request blood tests, hair or sweat analyses (for mineral deficiencies), and x-rays. The naturopathic treatment of hypertension usually involves diet and lifestyle advice, breathing exercises, skin brushing (to boost circulation), nutritional supplements, herbal remedies or homoeopathic medicines. You usually need at least four follow-up sessions of 30 minutes each.

the full-strength program day eight

Daily menu

- **Breakfast: home-made muesli (see page 100) with raspberries and shaved coconut**

- **Morning snack: a portion of superfood fruit (see day one)**

- **Lunch: low-fat cottage cheese mixed with chopped pears and Brazil nuts. Bowl of mixed salad leaves sprinkled with pumpkin seeds and Mediterranean herb oil (see page 168). Wholemeal roll. Fresh fruit**

- **Afternoon snack: a handful of almonds**

- **Dinner: salmon steak marinated in olive oil, lime juice and coriander, then grilled. Rocket leaves and pumpkin seeds drizzled with walnut oil. Brown rice. 40–50g (about 1½oz) bar dark chocolate**

- **Drinks: 570ml (1pt) semi-skimmed or skimmed milk. Freshly squeezed fruit/veg juice. Unlimited green/black or white tea, herbal tea and mineral water. 150ml (5fl oz) red wine or unsweetened red grape juice**

- **Supplements: see page 145**

From today I'd like you to meditate twice a day for 10–20 minutes each time. Start with 10 minutes twice a day and slowly build up to 15 or 20 minutes at each session. Choose whichever meditation you like for the second session.

Daily exercise routine

Do the first seven postures of the sun salutation (see days one to seven) when you get up, followed by the posture below. Walk briskly for 30–45 minutes or swim or cycle for 20 minutes. In the evening, unwind in corpse pose (see page 97) for 15 minutes.

Sun salutation – 8th posture

1 After the last pose, exhale and hold your breath. Lower yourself so your toes, chin, chest and knees touch the floor – your bottom stays in the air.

2 Relax. Breathe gently in and out. Keep your mind empty.

Meditation

Today you will do an advanced chakra meditation that both cleanses and re-energizes your chakras. You will need a small piece of amethyst, diamond or quartx. These crystals are associated with the crown chakra. Crystals have their own resonance that amplifies the power of meditation.

Chakra meditation with a crystal

1 Sit comfortably, holding the crystal in both hands on your lap. Visualize light or "white energy" moving from your base chakra up through your chakras to your crown chakra.

2 Imagine the light flowing from the crown of your head down through the crystal where it is amplified. Let the light flow back into the base of your spine and up through your chakras to form a continuous flowing wheel of light.

Avoid slips in motivation

Motivation can wane after a week of daily aerobic exercise. Keep varying your route, exercise with a friend, and check to see whether your blood pressure has come down.

!

day nine

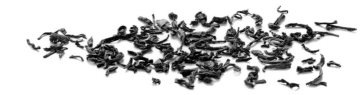

Daily menu

- **Breakfast: stuffed tomatoes (see page 165). Slice of wholemeal toast**

- **Morning snack: a portion of super-food fruit (see day one)**

- **Lunch: beetroot and tofu medley (see page 166). Bowl of mixed salad leaves sprinkled with walnuts, pumpkin seeds, chopped garlic, walnut oil and red wine vinegar. Low-fat bio yogurt with fresh fruit**

- **Afternoon snack: chocolate petit fours (see page 173)**

- **Dinner: Thai fish parcels (see page 171). Pak choi. Sweetcorn. Almond rice pudding (see page 172)**

- **Drinks: 570ml (1pt) semi-skimmed or skimmed milk. Freshly squeezed fruit/veg juice. Unlimited green/black or white tea, herbal tea and mineral water. 150ml (5fl oz) red wine or unsweetened red grape juice**

- **Supplements: see page 145**

The pak choi in tonight's dinner is a good source of carotenoids, calcium, magnesium, folic acid, vitamin C, vitamin K and potassium, making it ideal for hypertension. It can be added raw to salads, lightly steamed or used in stir-fries. Pak choi with green rather than white stems has a higher phytonutrient content.

Daily exercise routine

When you get up in the morning do the first eight postures of the sun salutation (see days one to eight) followed by the posture below. Walk briskly for 30–45 minutes during the day. Alternatively, swim or cycle for 20 minutes. In the evening, relax in corpse pose (see page 97) for 15 minutes.

Sun salutation – 9th posture

1 Following on from the last pose, let your bottom drop to the floor, lift your chest and stomach and curl your head back in cobra (see page 96).

2 Hold your breath, and stay in the pose for a few seconds, keeping your mind quiet, before starting to breathe gently in and out again.

Meditation

Today's meditation is based on a breathing exercise.

Breath meditation

1 Count how many breaths you take in a minute – it's normally about 12. You are going to try to reduce this to six breaths.

2 Breathe in slowly and deeply through your nose, then out through your mouth. As you inhale, imagine oxygen entering your body through the pores of your skin as well as through your nose so your breathing rate can slow down naturally. At first, try breathing in and out at the same rate – for example, inhale for 5 seconds and exhale for 5 seconds.

3 Now speed up your inhalations and slow your exhalations so you spend around 3 seconds breathing in, and 7 seconds breathing out.

4 Focus on emptying your lungs completely, and on keeping air flow continuous. Don't hold your breath between inhaling and exhaling. It takes practice to breathe at the slow rate of just six breaths per minute.

the full-strength program day ten

Daily menu

- **Breakfast: banana cinnamon porridge (see page 100) with coconut shavings**

- **Morning snack: a portion of superfood fruit (see day one)**

- **Lunch: almond and broccoli salad (see page 166). Bowl of mixed salad leaves sprinkled with pumpkin seeds, chopped garlic, walnut oil and red wine vinegar. Wholemeal roll. Low-fat bio yogurt with fresh fruit**

- **Afternoon snack: beetroot power juice (see page 173)**

- **Dinner: creamy mushroom cups (see page 168). Red rice. Broccoli. Baked apples (see page 173)**

- **Drinks: 570ml (1pt) semi-skimmed or skimmed milk. Freshly squeezed fruit/veg juice. Unlimited green/black or white tea, herbal tea and mineral water. 150ml (5fl oz) red wine or unsweetened red grape juice**

- **Supplements: see page 145**

Broccoli, in today's lunch, contains antioxidants and substances such as sulphoraphane that increase the production of antioxidant detoxi-fication enzymes (glutathiones) throughout the body. These reduce damage to arterial wall linings and help to combat both athero-sclerosis and hypertension. Lightly steam broccoli to retain maximum nutritional content.

Daily exercise routine

When you get up, do the first nine postures of the sun salutation (see days one to nine) followed by the posture below. Walk briskly for 30–45 minutes or swim or cycle for 20 minutes. In the evening, lie down in corpse pose (see page 97) for 15 minutes.

Sun salutation – 10th posture

1 Following on from the last pos-ture, breathe out and push up through your feet and hands, lifting your bottom high in the air and straightening your legs.

2 Your body should be in an inverted "V" shape. This is downward dog (see page 92). Tuck your chin into your chest, push your tailbone to the ceiling and hold your breath. Stay in the position for a few seconds. Keep your mind quiet.

Meditation

In today's meditation, I'd like you to focus on raising the temperature of one of your hands. Research using biofeedback machines (see page 45) shows that you can use the power of thought to increase blood circulation and temperature in one hand by as much as 5 to 10 degrees. If you can dilate your blood vessels in this way, it can help to lower blood pressure and stop tension headaches.

Body temperature meditation

1 Quietly focus on your dominant hand. Imagine it getting warmer. Direct all your attention to your hand and feel the glow spreading throughout your palm and fingers. Do this for at least 15 minutes.

2 Afterwards, place your hands against your cheeks to see if you can feel a temperature difference between them. Alternatively, use a forehead thermometer to measure the skin temperature of each palm.

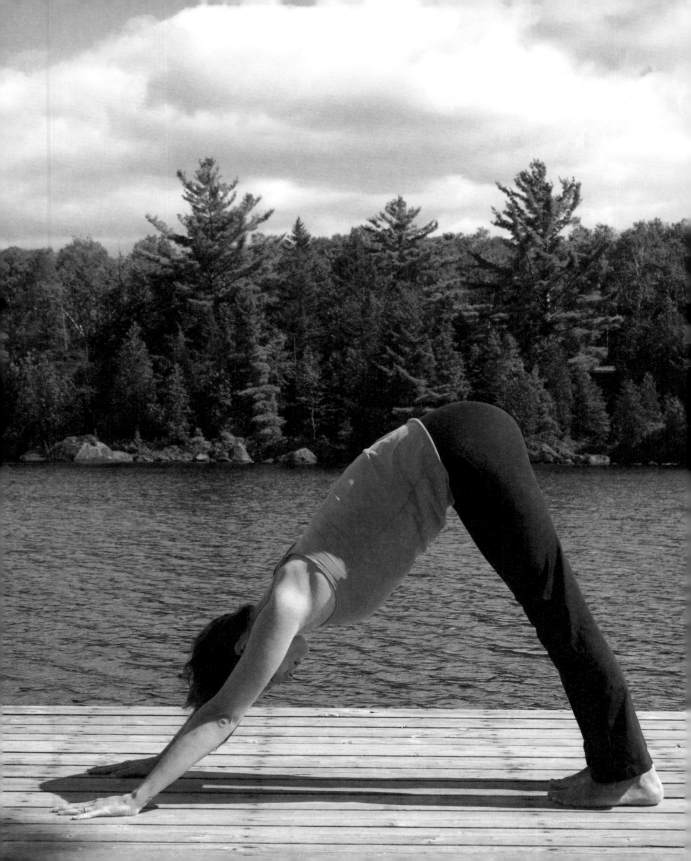

the full-strength program
day eleven

Daily menu

- **Breakfast: chopped figs, dates and apricots mixed with low-fat fromage frais. Slice of wholemeal, rye, soy or barley toast**

- **Morning snack: a portion of superfood fruit (see day one)**

- **Lunch: bowl of chopped avocado and low-fat buffalo mozzarella with tomatoes, walnuts and rocket, dressed with walnut oil and red wine vinegar. Low-fat bio yogurt with fresh fruit**

- **Afternoon snack: a handful of almonds**

- **Dinner: winter vegetable stew with rosemary (see page 170). Pears in red wine (see page 172)**

- **Drinks: 570ml (1pt) semi-skimmed or skimmed milk. Freshly squeezed fruit/veg juice. Unlimited green/black or white tea, herbal tea and mineral water. 150ml (5fl oz) red wine or unsweetened red grape juice**

- **Supplements: see page 145**

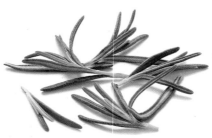

Daily exercise routine

Do the first 10 postures of the sun salutation (see days one to ten) this morning, followed by the posture below. Walk briskly for 30–45 minutes or swim or cycle for 20 minutes. In the evening, unwind by lying in the corpse pose (see page 97) for 15 minutes.

Sun salutation – 11th posture

1 Following on straight from the last posture, breathe in and take a big step forward with your left leg so your left foot falls in between your hands.
2 Still breathing in, raise your arms out and up in a wide circle, with your palms coming together above your head, fingers pointing up.
3 Look up at your hands and hold your breath, keeping your mind as empty as possible.

Meditation

Today I'd like you to focus on slowing your heart rate. Please note that if you are taking a beta-blocker drug you will not be able to influence your heart rate significantly

Heart-rate meditation

1 Spend 10 minutes sitting quietly, reading a book or listening to music. Take your pulse rate.
2 Now sit in quiet contemplation but, rather than focusing on a mantra, for example, focus on lowering your heart rate.
3 Imagine your heart beating in your chest. Send it mental signals to beat more slowly.
4 After 10 minutes, take your pulse rate again and see how much it has come down.

Watch your pulse

To help you with today's meditation you can buy a biofeedback device that provides a live readout of your heart rate on your home computer. You can watch your pulse rate fall as you meditate.

day twelve

Daily menu

- **Breakfast: home-made muesli (see page 100). Banana and walnuts**

- **Morning snack: a portion of superfood fruit (see day one)**

- **Lunch: green minestrone soup (see page 166). Wholemeal roll. Low-fat bio yogurt with fresh fruit**

- **Afternoon snack: raspberry almond smoothie (see page 173)**

- **Dinner: Mediterranean mackerel (see page 171). Wholemeal or hemp pasta. Broccoli. 40–50g (about 1½oz) bar dark chocolate**

- **Drinks: 570ml (1pt) semi-skimmed or skimmed milk. Freshly squeezed fruit/veg juice. Unlimited green/black or white tea, herbal tea and mineral water. 150ml (5fl oz) red wine or unsweetened red grape juice**

- **Supplements: see page 145**

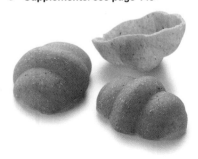

The meditations you are doing use principles borrowed from auto-genic training and biofeedback (see page 45). Research shows that people with high blood pressure can learn to reduce their blood pressure by 15.3/17.8mmHg during just three sessions of biofeedback training spread over a two-week period.

Daily exercise routine

When you get up, do the first 11 postures of the sun salutation (see days one to eleven) followed by the posture below. Walk briskly for 30–45 minutes during the day. Alternatively, swim or cycle for 20 minutes. In the evening, unwind by lying in the corpse pose (see page 97) for 15 minutes.

Sun salutation – 12th posture

1 Following straight on from the 11th posture, breathe out as you bring your right foot forward next to your left foot.

2 Grasp the backs of your ankles or calves (or as far down as feels comfortable).

3 Tuck your chin in and bend your elbows to pull your upper body gently in toward your legs.

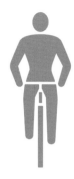

4 Breathe out and hold your breath for a few seconds while you stay in this pose, keeping your mind as quiet as possible.

Meditation

Today I'd like you to focus on lowering your blood pressure.

Blood pressure meditation

1 Spend 10 minutes sitting quietly, reading a book or listening to some music. Then take your blood pressure.

2 Sit in quiet contemplation – focus on bringing your blood pressure down.

3 Visualize your arteries and veins dilating, and imagine your pulse rate and breathing rate gradually becoming slower.

4 After 10 minutes, take your blood pressure again to discover by how much it has come down.

the full-strength program day thirteen

Daily menu

- **Breakfast: porridge with Brazil nuts and coconut shavings**

- **Morning snack: a portion of superfood fruit (see day one)**

- **Lunch: cheese, fruit and nut platter (see page 167). Bowl of mixed salad leaves sprinkled with Brazil nuts, pumpkin seeds, chopped garlic, walnut oil and red wine vinegar. Low-fat bio yogurt with fresh fruit**

- **Afternoon snack: chocolate florentines (see page 173)**

- **Dinner: lemon pork (see page 171). Spinach. Wholemeal or hemp pasta. Almond rice pudding (see page 172)**

- **Drinks: 570ml (1pt) semi-skimmed or skimmed milk. Freshly squeezed fruit/veg juice. Unlimited green/black or white tea, herbal tea and mineral water. 150ml (5fl oz) red wine or unsweetened red grape juice**

- **Supplements: see page 145**

Daily exercise routine

When you get up in the morning do the first 12 postures of the sun salutation (see days one to thirteen) followed by the posture below. Walk briskly for 30–45 minutes during the day or swim or cycle for 20 minutes. In the evening, lie down in corpse pose (see page 97) to unwind for 15 minutes.

Sun salutation – 13th posture

1 Following straight on from the last posture, breathe in and straighten up. As you straighten, bring your arms outward and up in a wide circle.

2 Bring your palms together over your head. Point your fingers up, look up at your hands and lengthen your spine.

3 Hold your breath and stay in this posture for a few seconds. Keep your mind as empty as possible.

Acupressure

I introduce you to a new home therapy today: acupressure. Massaging two acupressure points above the nape of your neck can help to bring blood pressure down.

These points are on the gall-bladder meridian and are called Gb20 (wind pool). To find them, place your thumbs on your ear-lobes and slide them back toward the base of your skull. They should fall into a small depression on either side of your neck vertebrae, about 2cm (1in) above your hair-line. Bend your head forward and back again to find them. Massage these points with firm thumb pressure for a minute. These points are also used to encourage the upward flow of energy through your chakras (see page 43).

Pumpkin seeds

Pumpkin seeds are a nutritious ingredient in today's lunch – and in many other lunches in this program. You can buy pumpkin seeds, but it's also easy to extract them from a pumpkin. Next time you eat pumpkin flesh, take out the seeds and either dry them in a warm oven for 3 hours, or toss them with olive oil and roast them for 10 minutes at 180°C/350°F/Gas 4.

day fourteen

Daily menu

- **Breakfast: cooked Sunday breakfast (see page 165). Slice of wholemeal, rye, soy or barley toast**

- **Morning snack: a portion of superfood fruit (see day one)**

- **Lunch: almond trout (see page 167). Bowl of mixed salad leaves sprinkled with coriander leaves, walnuts, pumpkin seeds, chopped garlic, walnut oil and red wine vinegar. Low-fat bio yogurt with fresh fruit**

- **Afternoon snack: beetroot power juice (see page 173)**

- **Dinner: chickpea curry (see page 170). Almond rice (see page 170). 40–50g (about 1½oz) bar dark chocolate**

- **Drinks: 570ml (1pt) semi-skimmed or skimmed milk. Freshly squeezed fruit/veg juice. Unlimited green/black or white tea, herbal tea and mineral water. 150ml (5fl oz) red wine or unsweetened red grape juice**

- **Supplements: see page 145**

Once you have learned today's final posture in the sun salutation, you will have a flowing sequence of postures that you can practise every morning. This ancient exercise regime will help you to concentrate and stay calm. According to yoga adepts, if you can fit in only one yoga exercise per day, it should be the sun salutation.

Daily exercise routine

When you get up in the morning do the first 13 postures of the sun salutation (see days one to thirteen) followed by the final posture below. Walk briskly for 30–45 minutes during the day. Alternatively, swim or cycle for 20 minutes. In the evening, unwind by lying down in the corpse pose (see page 97) for 15 minutes.

Sun salutation – 14th posture

1 Following straight on from the 13th posture, breathe out and bring your arms down to your sides in a flowing circle.

2 Bring your palms together in a prayer position in front of your chest. You have now completed a full round of the sun salutation.

Consulting an acupuncturist

I suggest that you end the program with a course of traditional Chinese acupuncture. To find an acupuncturist, see page 174. Acupuncture regulates the flow of qi energy in your body and can help to stabilize your blood pressure at a lower level. During a consultation, a practitioner takes your medical history, examines you and assesses the condition of your tongue, pulse and tan tien (the area below the navel). Sterile, disposable, slender needles are inserted into the skin over selected acupoints, to a depth of 4–25mm (⅟₈in). This should not be uncomfortable. Usually, between six and 12 needles are used, with points on the hands and feet most commonly selected. Needles may be left in position for as little as a few seconds, while others may be left for 30–60 minutes. Withdrawal of the needles at the end of the session is usually painless. A course of 12 acupuncture treatments, over a period of six weeks, can significantly lower raised blood pressure and the effects can last for nine months or more after the final treatment.

continuing the full-strength program

You have just finished two weeks on the full-strength program – well done! I now advise that you continue with the eating plan for a further two weeks. This way you will experience a month of healthy eating and be very familiar with the foods you need to shop for and eat every day. After a month you can then start to vary the foods you eat, and include some new recipes. The following information will help you plan your future on the full-strength program.

Your long-term diet

The diet you have followed in the full-strength plan is based on heart-friendly superfoods (see pages 56–59). Eating these superfoods on a regular basis means that you will significantly reduce your risk of coronary heart disease (see page 18). To continue with this diet:

● Eat at least five (preferably eight to 10) servings daily of fruit, vegetables/saladstuff, garlic, almonds, dark chocolate, red wine or red grape juice.
● Eat fish four times a week (though you can eat less than this if you continue to take garlic and omega-3 fish oil supplements).
● Include as many of the superfoods on pages 56–59 as possible in your daily diet. For example, blueberries, chickpeas, grapes, spinach and pomegranate.
● Eat mainly vegetarian and fish meals. Research suggests that hypertension is linked with a high intake of red and processed meat, whereas wholegrains, fruit, nuts, fish and milk (a rich source of beneficial calcium) have a protective effect on the cardiovascular system. For detailed advice on what to look for when choosing fish and shellfish, see page 130 of the moderate program.
● When you do eat meat, choose poulty or non-fatty cuts of red meat such as lean pork.

Recipes Explore fish-based and vegetarian recipes – you will find delicious recipe suggestions at www.naturalhealthguru.co.uk. You can post your own favourite recipes there for other followers of the full-strength program to try. Bear the following points in mind when you are choosing recipes and cooking:

● Look for recipes that include superfoods such as red wine. Cooking with red wine removes excess alcohol, while retaining useful amounts of antioxidants.
● Include garlic in savoury dishes, even if the original recipe doesn't include it.
● Replace salt in recipes with freshly ground

Regular blood tests

If your cholesterol, triglyceride and homocysteine levels are in the optimum range, you need to have them checked annually. If they are raised above optimal, however (or below optimum in the case of good HDL-cholesterol), you may wish to have the non-optimal values assessed every three to six months.

pepper and handfuls of freshly chopped herbs.
- Replace cream with yogurt or fromage frais. For tips on how to use yogurt in cooking, see page 98.

Your long-term supplement regime

Continue taking the recommended supplements for the full-strength program (see page 145) long term. Findings from numerous studies back their use at this high level for significant effects on your blood pressure and future health. However, do not increase the doses further without specific, individual advice from a qualified nutritional therapist, naturopath or doctor. If, up until now, you have taken only the supplements in the recommended list, think about taking one or more of the supplements in the optional list for additional benefits. Full details of each supplement, including updates on latest research findings, are available at www.naturalhealthguru.co.uk

Your exercise routine

Continue with at least 45 minutes of aerobic exercise per day: brisk walking, cycling or swimming are ideal. If you don't already belong to a gym, think about joining one – a personal trainer will give you individually tailored advice, help to motivate you and provide suggestions for improving your muscular fitness as well as your aerobic fitness. Continue to perform the sun salutation every morning when you get up and spend 15 minutes in the corpse pose (see page 97) to wind down at the end of each day. If you enjoy the yoga, consider joining a class or receiving one-to-one tuition.

Your therapy program

The full-strength program has introduced you to a variety of advanced meditation practices. Continue meditating for at least 20 minutes per day, ideally on two occasions: once in the morning and once in the evening, using whichever of the meditation techniques you find most helpful. You can also attend meditation classes to receive formal instruction from a teacher (read about different types of meditation on page 45). If you found their interventions helpful, continue to consult the therapists – the naturopath and acupuncturist. Other complementary therapies to consider include biofeedback and autogenic training.

Monitoring your blood pressure

While continuing with the full-strength program, I suggest you monitor your blood pressure on a weekly basis, at the same time of day, unless your doctor has asked you to check it more frequently. Keep a record of your blood pressure measurements in a chart such as the one on page 77. This will give you an instant visual indication of whether your blood pressure is going down (which I would expect during this program), staying the same or going up.

If your blood pressure is consistently below 130/80mmHg, well done. The full-strength program has had the desired effect and, to consolidate the benefits, you should continue it long term. If you are taking prescribed anti-hypertensive medication, your doctor may consider lowering the dose or number of anti-hypertensive drugs you are taking, if he or she feels it's appropriate. This is not something you should do on your own without your doctor's supervision, however. The dose of some anti-hypertensive drugs needs to be reduced slowly to prevent any rebound effects.

If your blood pressure is consistently between 130/80mmHg and 140/90mmHg, seek advice from your doctor or naturopath to see if you can bring it down to below 130/80mmHg. Although a blood pressure of less than 140/90mmHg is an acceptable target, a level of less than 130/80mmHg is ideal for long-term health, especially if you also have diabetes or kidney problems. If your blood pressure is consistently above 140/90mmHg, see your doctor for individual advice.

breakfast recipes

herrings in oatmeal

serves 4

4 small herrings, gutted, descaled, head
   and backbone removed
4 tbsp semi-skimmed cow's, almond,
   rice or soy milk
4 tbsp coarse oatmeal
2 tbsp olive oil
Freshly squeezed juice of 1 lime
1 large handful watercress
Freshly ground black pepper

1 Dip the herrings in the milk and
   then roll in the oatmeal. Season
   with black pepper.
2 Heat the oil in a pan. Add the
   herrings and fry over gentle
   heat for about 10 minutes on
   each side. Sprinkle each fish
   with a little lime juice and serve
   on a bed of watercress.

windward islands trout

serves 4

4 trout fillets, about 150g/5½oz each
2 small bananas, peeled and cut in half
   lengthways
Freshly squeezed juice of 1 orange
Grated zest and freshly squeezed juice
   of 1 unwaxed lemon
1 handful watercress, rinsed and
   drained
1 handful fresh flat-leaf parsley, roughly
   chopped
Freshly ground black pepper

1 Preheat the oven to
   180°C/350°F/Gas 4.
2 Arrange the trout in a single
   layer in a baking dish. Lay half
   a banana along each fillet and
   pour over the citrus juice and
   zest. Bake for 20 minutes, or
   until the fish is cooked through.

3 Season with black pepper and
   serve on a bed of watercress
   sprinkled with the parsley.

blueberry and almond mousse

serves 4

400g/14oz/2½ cups blueberries
300g/10½oz silken tofu
100g/3½oz/¾ cup blanched almonds,
   roughly chopped

1 Reserve a few blueberries for
   serving, then place the remainder in a blender with the tofu
   and process until smooth.
2 Divide between 4 glass serving bowls. Sprinkle over the
   chopped almonds, top with the
   reserved blueberries and serve.

below: windward islands trout

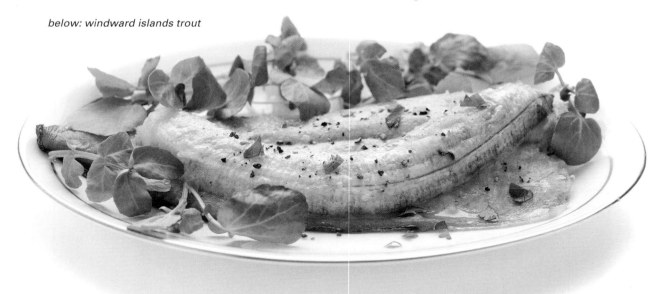

cooked sunday breakfast

. . . .

serves 4

4 mushrooms, cut in half
4 medium tomatoes, cut in half
4 small courgettes, cut in half
   lengthways
1 red pepper, deseeded and cut into
   8 pieces
1 yellow pepper, deseeded and cut into
   8 pieces
4 tbsp olive oil
4 handfuls spinach leaves, washed
Freshly ground black pepper
4 slices wholemeal toast, to serve

1 Preheat the grill to medium-hot.
2 Put the mushrooms, tomatoes, courgettes and peppers on a baking sheet and drizzle with the oil. Put under the grill and cook until the vegetables are just tender. Meanwhile, cook the spinach leaves in a steamer until they wilt.
3 Divide the grilled vegetables and spinach between four warm serving plates. Season with black pepper and serve with the toast.

right: stuffed tomatoes

stuffed tomatoes

. . . .

serves 4

4 beef tomatoes
1 shallot, finely chopped
2 garlic cloves, crushed
12 fresh basil leaves, torn
1 handful fresh parsley, chopped
175g/6oz mushrooms, sliced
1 handful grated mozzarella cheese
   (optional)
Freshly ground black pepper
4 slices wholemeal or rye toast,
   to serve

1 Preheat the oven to 180°C/350°F/Gas 4.
2 Slice the tops off the tomatoes. Scoop out the insides and mix with the shallot, garlic, herbs and mushrooms. Season with pepper. Stuff the tomatoes with the mixture. Top with the cheese (if using) and replace the tomato tops. Bake for 15 minutes. Serve with toast.

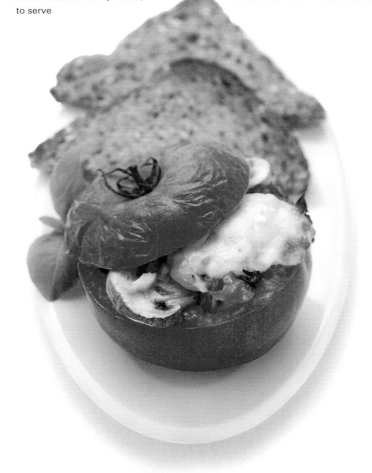

lunch recipes

green minestrone

serves 4

1 tbsp olive oil
1 onion, chopped
1 leek, chopped
4 garlic cloves, crushed
1l/35fl oz/4 cups vegetable stock (see page 109) or water
100g/3½oz green lasagne sheets, broken into bite-sized pieces
100g/3½oz broccoli florets
100g/3½oz/¾ cup green peas, fresh or frozen
100g/3½oz shredded green leaves, such as spinach, kale, savoy cabbage or pak choi
1 courgette, finely chopped
1 handful fresh basil leaves, shredded
Freshly ground black pepper

1 Heat the oil in a large frying pan. Add the onion, leek and garlic and cook over a medium heat until soft. Pour in the vegetable stock and bring to the boil. Add the green pasta pieces and cook for 5 minutes.

2 Add the broccoli, peas, green leaves and courgette and simmer gently for another 3 minutes. Stir in the basil leaves, season with black pepper and serve.

almond and broccoli salad

serves 4

450g/1lb broccoli florets
4 tbsp walnut or extra virgin olive oil
3 tbsp lemon juice
1 garlic clove, crushed
2 sprigs oregano or thyme, leaves chopped
Freshly ground black pepper
4 large spring onions, roughly chopped
100g/3½oz/scant 1 cup flaked almonds, lightly toasted

1 Plunge the broccoli into a pan of boiling water. Return to the boil and cook for 1 minute. Drain and then plunge into cold water.

2 Put the oil, lemon juice, garlic and oregano in a small bowl and mix well. Season with black pepper.

3 Toss the broccoli, spring onions and almonds in a large serving bowl. Pour over the oil and lemon mixture and serve.

beetroot and tofu medley

serves 4

250g/9oz firm tofu, cubed
250g/9oz cooked baby beetroot, peeled and cubed
1 small red onion, thinly sliced
1 ripe avocado, peeled, stoned and flesh roughly chopped
Freshly squeezed juice of 1 lime
2 tbsp walnut or extra virgin olive oil
2 tsp wholegrain mustard
250g/9oz mixed baby salad leaves
Freshly ground black pepper

1 Mix the tofu, beetroot, onion and avocado in a bowl and set aside.

2 Put the lime juice, oil and mustard in a screw-top jar and shake until thoroughly mixed Pour over the tofu and beetroot mixture and toss well.

3 Put the salad leaves in a serving bowl and top with the tofu and beetroot mixture. Season with pepper and serve.

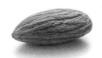

almond trout

serves 4

4 trout fillets, about 200g/7oz each
4 tbsp semi-skimmed cow's, almond,
  rice or soy milk
4 tbsp ground almonds
2 tbsp olive oil
4 medium tomatoes, cut in half
4 tbsp flaked almonds, lightly toasted
Freshly ground black pepper

1 Dip the trout in the milk and
  roll in the ground almonds until
  evenly coated. Set aside.
2 Heat the oil in a large frying
  pan. Add the tomatoes and
  trout and cook over gentle heat
  for about 4 minutes on each
  side, until the fish is cooked.
3 Arrange the trout and tomatoes
  on four warm serving plates.
  Season with pepper, sprinkle
  with the almonds and serve.

cheese, fruit and nut platter

serves 4

250g/9oz mixed salad leaves
2 handfuls watercress
2 oranges, peeled, pith removed and
  thinly sliced

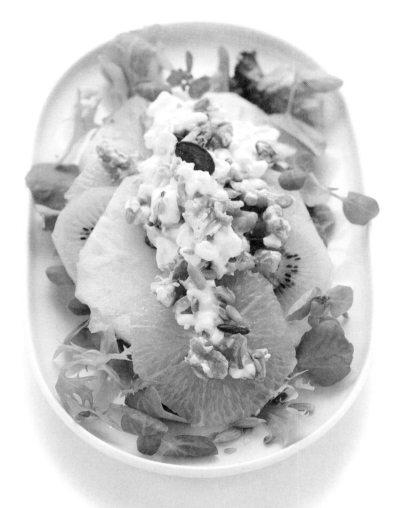

cheese, fruit and nut platter

1 small pineapple, peeled, cored and
  thinly sliced
1 kiwi fruit, peeled and thinly sliced
250g/9oz cottage cheese
100g/3½oz/1 cup walnuts
100g/3½oz/scant 1 cup mixed seeds,
  such as linseed, sunflower, pumpkin
  and sesame

1 Put the salad leaves and watercress on a large serving dish
  and arrange the fruit on top.
2 Mix the cottage cheese,
  walnuts and seeds in a bowl.
  Pile this mixture on top of the
  fruit and serve.

dinner recipes

creamy mushroom cups

• • • • • • • • • • • • • • • • •

serves 4

1 shallot, finely chopped
1 handful fresh parsley, roughly
    chopped
150g/5½oz silken tofu
Grated zest and freshly squeezed juice
    of 1 unwaxed lemon
Freshly ground black pepper
12 small mushrooms, stalks removed
1 tsp paprika
1 handful mixed salad leaves, to serve

1　Put the shallot, parsley and tofu
    in a bowl and mash together to
    form a paste. Stir in the lemon
    juice and zest and season with
    black pepper.
2　Put the mushrooms, hollow-
    side up on a serving platter.
    Pile the tofu mixture into the
    mushrooms, sprinkle each one
    with a little paprika and serve
    with the salad leaves.

mediterranean herb oil

• •

600ml/1pt/2½ cups extra virgin
    olive oil
12 black peppercorns
12 green peppercorns
12 fennel seeds
12 coriander seeds
2 sprigs rosemary
2 sprigs thyme
2 sprigs tarragon
2 sprigs oregano
2 bay leaves
2 red chillies, scored lengthways

1　Put all the ingredients in a clear
    wine bottle. Cork to form a
    tight seal. Shake well.
2　Put in a warm place, such as a
    sunny windowsill, and leave for
    at least 2 weeks, shaking and
    turning the bottle every day.
    Use as required.

oriental tofu stir-fry

• •

serves 4

1 tbsp olive oil
4 garlic cloves, crushed
5cm/2in piece fresh ginger, peeled and
    grated
400g/14oz firm tofu, cut into 2cm/¾in
    cubes
200g/7oz broccoli florets
200g/7oz mangetout or sugarsnap peas
200g/7oz pak choi, coarsely shredded
200g/7oz bean sprouts
1l/35fl oz/4 cups vegetable stock (see
    page 109)
Freshly ground black pepper
2 tbsp flaked almonds
1 handful fresh coriander leaves,
    roughly chopped

1　Swirl the olive oil in a hot frying
    pan or wok. Add the garlic and
    ginger and stir-fry over high
    heat for 1 minute. Toss in the
    tofu, broccoli, mangetout, pak
    choi and bean sprouts and stir-
    fry for another 3 minutes.
2　Pour in the stock, bring to the
    boil and simmer for 2 minutes.
    Season with pepper, sprinkle
    with the flaked almonds and
    coriander leaves and serve.

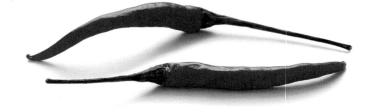

right: oriental tofu stir-fry

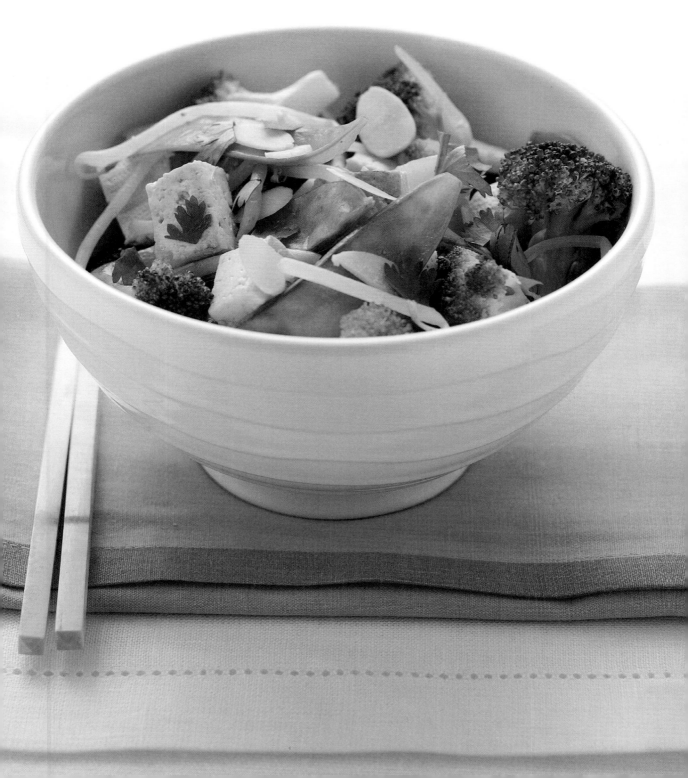

almond rice

serves 4

½ tbsp olive oil
1 onion, chopped
2 garlic cloves
200g/7oz/1 cup long-grain brown or
    red rice
1 handful raisins
600ml/1pt/2½ cups vegetable stock (see
    page 109)
1 handful flaked almonds
1 handful fresh flat-leaf parsley, roughly
    chopped

1 Heat the oil in a pan. Add the
   onion and garlic and cook over
   medium heat until soft. Add the
   rice and stir-fry for 1 minute.
   Meanwhile, heat the stock in
   a separate pan.

2 Stir the raisins into the rice,
   pour over the hot stock and
   bring to the boil. Lower the
   heat, cover and simmer gently,
   stirring occasionally, for about
   30 minutes, or until the rice
   is tender and all the liquid has
   been absorbed. If the rice
   needs further cooking, add a
   little more stock or water and
   continue until the rice is tender.

3 Remove the pan from the heat.
   Fold in the almonds and parsley
   and serve hot or cold.

chickpea curry

serves 4

1 tbsp extra virgin olive oil
1 onion, chopped
4 garlic cloves, crushed
5cm/2in piece fresh ginger, peeled and
    grated
6 tsp coriander seeds, crushed or
    ground
3 tsp cumin seeds, ground
1–2 red chillies, deseeded and finely
    chopped
1 large tomato, skinned, deseeded and
    chopped
125g/4½oz mushrooms, sliced
400g/14oz tin chickpeas, drained
200ml/7fl oz/¾ cup coconut milk
Freshly squeezed juice of 1 lime
1–2 handfuls fresh coriander leaves,
    roughly chopped
1 handful flaked almonds, lightly
    toasted
Freshly ground black pepper

1 Heat the oil in a pan. Add the
   onion and cook over medium
   heat for about 3 minutes, until
   soft. Add the garlic, ginger,
   coriander and cumin seeds and
   chillies and stir-fry for another
   3 minutes. Add the tomato and
   mushrooms and cook for a
   further 5 minutes.

2 Add the chickpeas, coconut
   milk, lime juice and 1 handful of
   coriander. Simmer for 10 minutes. Season with pepper and
   sprinkle with the almonds and
   another handful of coriander.

winter vegetable
stew with rosemary

serves 4

2 butternut squash, or half a large
    pumpkin, peeled, deseeded and
    chopped
1l/35fl oz/4 cups vegetable stock (see
    page 109) or water
1 onion, chopped
1 bay leaf
1 handful rosemary sprigs
1 tbsp extra virgin olive oil
2 leeks, chopped
4 garlic cloves, crushed
1 parsnip, chopped
2 sweet potatoes, chopped
200g/7oz tin butter beans, drained
Freshly ground black pepper

1 Put half the squash in a pan
   with the stock, onion, bay leaf
   and most of the rosemary (set
   aside a few sprigs to serve).
   Bring to the boil, lower the heat
   and leave to simmer for 30
   minutes. Remove the bay leaf,
   allow to cool a little, then purée
   in a blender. Set aside.

2 Heat the oil in a clean pan. Add
   the leeks and garlic and stir-fry
   until soft. Add the remaining
   squash, parsnip and sweet
   potatoes and stir-fry for a
   further 5 minutes.

3 Stir in the butter beans and
   puréed squash. Leave to
   simmer for 30 minutes. Season
   with pepper and serve with
   rosemary sprigs.

lemon pork

serves 4

1 shallot, chopped
4 garlic cloves
1 tbsp olive oil
4 lean pork fillets, about 175g/6oz
    each, cut into cubes
3 tsp cumin seeds, ground
3 tsp coriander seeds, ground
300ml/10½fl oz/3 glasses light red
    wine, such as Beaujolais
1 lemon, thinly sliced
Freshly ground black pepper

1 Cook the shallot and garlic in the oil. Add the pork and cumin and coriander seeds and stir gently to brown the meat.

2 Add half the wine and simmer gently for 25 minutes. Stir in the lemon and remaining wine. Season with pepper and serve.

mackerel and cucumber in wine

serves 4

½ small cucumber, sliced
4 mackerel fillets, about 150g/5½oz each
1 handful fresh dill or flat-leaf
    parsley, roughly chopped
100ml/3½fl oz/1 glass dry white wine
Freshly ground black pepper

1 Preheat the oven to 180°C/350°F/Gas 4.

2 Line a dish with the cucumber. Add the other ingredients, cover and bake for 30 minutes.

mediterranean mackerel

serves 4

½ tbsp olive oil
1 onion, chopped
2 garlic cloves, chopped
350g/12oz ripe tomatoes, skinned,
    deseeded and chopped
Freshly squeezed juice and grated zest
    of 1 large unwaxed lemon
1 bay leaf
4 mackerel fillets, about 150g/5½oz each
Freshly ground black pepper
1 handful fresh flat-leaf parsley, roughly
    chopped

1 Preheat the grill to hot.

2 Heat the oil in a pan. Add the onion and garlic and cook over medium heat for 5 minutes, until soft. Add the tomatoes, lemon juice and zest, and bay leaf, cover and leave to simmer gently for about 15 minutes.

3 Meanwhile, put the mackerel fillets in a single layer on a baking sheet, season with pepper and grill for about 10 minutes, turning halfway through the cooking time.

4 Put the grilled mackerel on four warm serving plates. Top each one with some of the hot tomato sauce, sprinkle with parsley and serve.

thai fish parcels

serves 4

1 lemongrass stalk, peeled and finely
    chopped
4 garlic cloves, crushed
2 shallots, chopped
Freshly squeezed juice and grated zest
    of 1 unwaxed lime
1½ tbsp extra virgin or olive oil
1 green chilli, deseeded and chopped
1 red chilli, deseeded and chopped
1 handful fresh coriander leaves,
    roughly chopped
4 sea bass fillets, about 200g/7oz each

1 Preheat the oven to 180°C/350°F/Gas 4.

2 Put the lemongrass, garlic, shallots, lime juice and zest, oil, chillies and coriander leaves in a blender and process to form a paste.

3 Lay each fish fillet in the centre of a piece of foil, large enough to wrap around it to form a parcel. Spread one quarter of the spicy mixture over the top of each piece of fish and fold up the foil to form four well-sealed parcels. Put the parcels on a baking sheet and bake in the hot oven for 15 minutes.

dessert recipes

almond rice pudding

serves 4

200g/7oz/1 cup long-grain brown rice
1l/35fl oz/4 cups almond milk
1 cinnamon stick
1 handful flaked almonds
1 handful dried dates, chopped
  (optional)

1 Put the rice, almond milk and
   cinnamon stick in a pan and
   bring to the boil. Lower the
   heat, cover and leave to
   simmer gently for 40 minutes,
   stirring occasionally, until the
   rice is tender and all the liquid
   is absorbed.
2 Serve hot or cold, sprinkled
   with the flaked almonds and
   chopped dates, if using.

almond chocolate cups

serves 4

100g/3½oz dark chocolate, plus extra
  grated chocolate to serve
250g/9oz silken tofu
1 handful ground almonds
1 handful flaked almonds

1 Melt the chocolate. Using a
   pastry brush, paint the chocolate over the sides and bases
   of four paper muffin cases,
   so each has a thick chocolate
   lining. Put in the fridge. When
   hard, peel off the paper case.
2 Process the tofu and ground
   almonds in a blender. Fill the
   chocolate cups with this mixture, then chill in the fridge.
   Serve sprinkled with the
   flaked almonds and grated
   chocolate.

pears in red wine

serves 4

4 firm dessert pears
1 cinnamon stick
300ml/½pt/3 glasses fruity red wine,
  such as Beaujolais
3 tsp clear honey (optional)
Low-fat fromage frais, to serve

1 Preheat the oven to
   180°C/350°F/Gas 4.
2 Halve each pear lengthways
   and scoop out the core. Thinly
   pare away the skin. Put the
   pears in an oven-proof dish
   with the cinnamon stick. Pour
   over the red wine and carefully
   stir in the honey, if using.
3 Cover the dish with foil and
   bake for 20 minutes. Remove
   from the oven, turn the pears
   over, re-cover with foil, then
   return to the oven and cook for
   a further 20 minutes until the
   pears are tender. Serve hot or
   cold with the fromage frais.

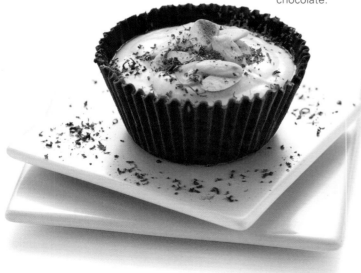

almond chocolate cups

bites, snacks and drinks

baked apples

serves 4

4 Bramley apples
1 handful flaked almonds
1 handful walnuts, roughly chopped
1 small handful raisins
Freshly squeezed juice and zest of
   1 unwaxed lemon
60ml/2fl oz/½ glass white wine
Low-fat fromage frais, to serve

1 Preheat the oven to
   180°C/350°F/Gas 4.
2 Cut the cores out of the apples,
   leaving them whole. With a
   sharp knife, cut just through
   the skin around the middle of
   each fruit. Stand the apples
   upright in a baking dish.
3 Mix together the almonds,
   walnuts, raisins and lemon
   juice and zest in a small bowl.
   Stuff a little of this mixture into
   the hollow in the centre of each
   apple. Pour a little wine over
   each apple.
4 Bake for 30 minutes, basting
   occasionally with the juices,
   until the apples are tender.
   Serve hot with fromage frais.

toasted almonds with seeds

serves 4

1 handful blanched almonds
1 handful pumpkin seeds
1 handful sunflower seeds
1 handful linseed seeds
1 handful raisins (optional)

1 Toast the almonds and the
   seeds in a dry pan for a few
   seconds, stirring until they turn
   golden brown.
2 Let the nuts and seeds cool in
   a shallow dish. Mix in the
   raisins, if using, and serve.

raspberry almond smoothie

serves 4

600ml/1pt/2½ cups almond milk
4 handfuls fresh raspberries
2 handfuls crushed ice
Fresh mint leaves, to serve

1 Put all the ingredients, except
   the mint, in a blender and
   process until smooth.
2 Pour into four tall serving
   glasses. Top with the mint
   leaves and serve immediately.

chocolate petit fours

serves 4

100g/3½oz seedless black grapes
100g/3½oz/⅔ cup Brazil nuts
100g/3½oz dark chocolate, melted

1 Dip each grape and nut into the
   chocolate. Chill until set.

chocolate florentines

serves 4

200g/7oz dark chocolate, melted
1 handful flaked almonds
1 handful dried cranberries
Grated zest of 1 unwaxed lemon

1 Drop small spoonfuls of chocolate onto greaseproof paper.
   Top each chocolate round
   with almonds, cranberries and
   lemon zest. Chill until set.

beetroot power juice

serves 4

450g/1lb raw beetroot, roughly chopped
4 carrots, peeled and roughly chopped
4 oranges, peeled and roughly chopped
1 handful crushed ice

1 Juice the beetroot, carrots and
   oranges. Mix. Serve with ice.

resources

Visit

www.naturalhealthguru.co.uk for more information, medical references and to post questions or comments about the Natural Health Guru programs.

Blood pressure

- American Heart Association
  www.americanheart.org

- American Hypertension Society
  www.ash-us.org

- Blood Pressure Association (UK)
  www.bpassoc.org.uk

- British Heart Foundation
  www.bhf.org.uk

- British Hypertension Society
  www.bhsoc.org

- Canadian Hypertension Society
  www.hypertension.ca

- European Society of Hypertension
  www.eshonline.org

- High Blood Pressure Research Council of Australia
  www.hbprca.com.au

- National Heart Foundation of Australia
  www.heartfoundation.com.au

Salt

- Consensus Action on Salt and Health (CASH)
  www.hyp.ac.uk/cash

Aromatherapy

- Australia: International Federation of Aromatherapists
  www.ifa.org.au

- UK: International Federation of Professional Aromatherapists
  www.ifparoma.org

- US: National Association of Holistic Aromatherapists
  www.naha.org

Acupuncture

- Australian Acupuncture and Oriental Medicine Alliance www.aomalliance.org

- American Association of Oriental Medicine
  www.aaom.org

- British Acupuncture Council
  www.acupuncture.org.uk

- British Medical Acupuncture Society
  www.medical-acupuncture.co.uk

- Chinese Medicine and Acupuncture Association of Canada
  www.cmaac.ca

Herbal medicine

- International Register of Consultant Herbalists and Homeopaths
  www.irch.org

- UK National Institute of Medical Herbalists
  www.nimh.org.uk

* National Herbalists Association of Australia
  www.nhaa.org.au

* American Herbalists Guild
  www.americanherbalistsguild.com

* Ontario Herbalists Association
  www.herbalists.on.ca

Homeopathy

* Australian Homeopathic Association
  www.homeopathyoz.org

* American Institute of Homeopathy
  www.homeopathyusa.org

* Canadian National United Professional Association of Trained Homeopaths
  www.nupath.org

* Faculty of Homeopathy (UK)
  www.trusthomeopathy.org

* International Register of Consultant Herbalists and Homeopaths
  www.irch.org

Naturopathy

* American Association of Naturopathic Physicians
  www.naturopathic.org

* Australian Naturopathic Practitioners Association
  www.anpa.asn.au

* British Naturopathic Association
  www.naturopaths.org.uk

* Canadian Association of Naturopathic Medicine
  www.ccnm.edu

Reflexology

* Association of Reflexologists (UK)
  www.aor.org.uk

* British Reflexology Association
  www.britreflex.co.uk

* Reflexology Association of America
  www.reflexology-usa.org

* Reflexology Association of Australia
  www.reflexology.org.au

* Reflexology Association of Canada
  www.reflexologycanada.ca

Yoga

* British Wheel of Yoga
  www.bwy.org.uk

* American Yoga Association
  www.americanyogaassociation.org

* Canadian Yoga Alliance
  www.canadianyogicalliance.com

* Yoga Centers Australia
  www.yoga-centers-directory.net

index

acknowledgments

The publisher would like to thank the following photographic libraries for permission to reproduce their material. Every care has been taken to trace copyright holders. However, if we have omitted anyone we apologize and will, if informed, make corrections to any future edition.

page 34 Noah Clayton / The Image Bank / Getty Images; **83** Jutta Klee / Corbis; **117** John Kelly / The Image Bank / Getty Images; **125** Noah Clayton / The Image Bank / Getty Images; **149** Caroline von Tuempling / Iconica / Getty Images; **157** Ron Levine / Riser / Getty Images

Author's acknowledgments

I would like to thank my husband, Richard, who willingly provided invaluable back up and support during those long hours of research and writing. I would also like to thank everyone who has helped in bringing this book to fruition, including Grace Cheetham at Duncan Baird, Judy Barratt and Kesta Desmond – who ensured consistency throughout – and, of course, my inimitable agent, Mandy Little.